TRACK
FOOD & WATER
EXERCISE
SLEEP

FOR THE NEXT 60 DAYS - YOU CAN DO IT!

RECORD YOUR GOALS

NAME: _____.

WHAT DO YOU WANT TO ACHIEVE OVER THE NEXT 60 DAYS?:

TRACK YOUR PROGRESS

RECORD YOUR MEASUREMENTS BEFORE YOU START, MIDWAY THROUGH, THEN AGAIN AT 60 DAYS

	START	30 DAYS	60 DAYS
WEIGHT:	-----------	-----------	-----------
UPPER ARM:	-----------	-----------	-----------
CHEST:	-----------	-----------	-----------
STOMACH:	-----------	-----------	-----------
HIPS	-----------	-----------	-----------
WAIST:	-----------	-----------	-----------
BUTT:	-----------	-----------	-----------
THIGH:	-----------	-----------	-----------
CALF:	-----------	-----------	-----------

NOTES:

DAY 1

M T W T F S S

DAY: _____ MONTH: _____ YEAR: _____

BREAKFAST	CALORIES	CARBS (g)	FAT (g)	PROTEIN (g)	FIBER (g)	SUGAR (g)	SODIUM (mg)
MORNING SNACK							
TOTAL:							

LUNCH	CALORIES	CARBS (g)	FAT (g)	PROTEIN (g)	FIBER (g)	SUGAR (g)	SODIUM (mg)
MIDDAY SNACK							
TOTAL:							

DINNER	CALORIES	CARBS (g)	FAT (g)	PROTEIN (g)	FIBER (g)	SUGAR (g)	SODIUM (mg)
EVENING SNACK							
TOTAL:							

DAILY TOTAL:							

WATER INTAKE:

☐ ☐ ☐ ☐ ☐ ☐ ☐ ☐ ☐ ☐
1 OZ 2 OZ 3 OZ 4 OZ 5 OZ 6 OZ 7 OZ 8 OZ 9 OZ 10 OZ

TYPE OF EXERCISE/ACTIVITY	HOW LONG?	INTENSITY	CALORIES BURNED
TOTAL CALORIES BURNED:			

SLEEP TRACKER:

○ ○ ○ ○ ○ ○ ○ ○ ○ ○
1 hr 2 hrs 3 hrs 4 hrs 5 hrs 6 hrs 7 hrs 8 hrs 9 hrs 10 hrs

QUALITY OF SLEEP
☆ ☆ ☆ ☆ ☆

Describe your mood throughout the day. Note in particular the times when you felt 'high' or 'low'. What food/activity affected your mood and/or overall well-being today?

_____

_____

_____

What did you crave today? When did you crave it, and why?
What did you do to manage your cravings throughout the day? Were you successful?

_____

_____

_____

Additional notes/observations i.e. weight, muscle tone, shape, setbacks, motivation etc.

_____

_____

_____

How can you make tomorrow even better?

_____

_____

_____

DAY 2

BREAKFAST	CALORIES	CARBS (g)	FAT (g)	PROTEIN (g)	FIBER (g)	SUGAR (g)	SODIUM (mg)
MORNING SNACK							
TOTAL:							

LUNCH	CALORIES	CARBS (g)	FAT (g)	PROTEIN (g)	FIBER (g)	SUGAR (g)	SODIUM (mg)
MIDDAY SNACK							
TOTAL:							

DINNER	CALORIES	CARBS (g)	FAT (g)	PROTEIN (g)	FIBER (g)	SUGAR (g)	SODIUM (mg)
EVENING SNACK							
TOTAL:							
DAILY TOTAL:							

WATER INTAKE:

☐ ☐ ☐ ☐ ☐ ☐ ☐ ☐ ☐ ☐
1 OZ 2 OZ 3 OZ 4 OZ 5 OZ 6 OZ 7 OZ 8 OZ 9 OZ 10 OZ

TYPE OF EXERCISE/ACTIVITY	HOW LONG?	INTENSITY	CALORIES BURNED
		TOTAL CALORIES BURNED:	

SLEEP TRACKER:

○ ○ ○ ○ ○ ○ ○ ○ ○ ○
1 hr 2 hrs 3 hrs 4 hrs 5 hrs 6 hrs 7 hrs 8 hrs 9 hrs 10 hrs

QUALITY OF SLEEP
☆ ☆ ☆ ☆ ☆

Describe your mood throughout the day. Note in particular the times when you felt 'high' or 'low'. What food/activity affected your mood and/or overall well-being today?

_____

_____

_____

_____

What did you crave today? When did you crave it, and why?
What did you do to manage your cravings throughout the day? Were you successful?

_____

_____

_____

_____

Additional notes/observations i.e. weight, muscle tone, shape, setbacks, motivation etc.

_____

_____

_____

_____

How can you make tomorrow even better?

_____

_____

_____

DAY 3

DAY: _____   MONTH: _____   YEAR: _____

BREAKFAST	CALORIES	CARBS (g)	FAT (g)	PROTEIN (g)	FIBER (g)	SUGAR (g)	SODIUM (mg)
MORNING SNACK							
TOTAL:							

LUNCH	CALORIES	CARBS (g)	FAT (g)	PROTEIN (g)	FIBER (g)	SUGAR (g)	SODIUM (mg)
MIDDAY SNACK							
TOTAL:							

DINNER	CALORIES	CARBS (g)	FAT (g)	PROTEIN (g)	FIBER (g)	SUGAR (g)	SODIUM (mg)
EVENING SNACK							
TOTAL:							

DAILY TOTAL:							

WATER INTAKE:

☐ ☐ ☐ ☐ ☐ ☐ ☐ ☐ ☐ ☐
1 OZ   2 OZ   3 OZ   4 OZ   5 OZ   6 OZ   7 OZ   8 OZ   9 OZ   10 OZ

TYPE OF EXERCISE/ACTIVITY	HOW LONG?	INTENSITY	CALORIES BURNED
	TOTAL CALORIES BURNED:		

SLEEP TRACKER:

○ ○ ○ ○ ○ ○ ○ ○ ○ ○
1 hr 2 hrs 3 hrs 4 hrs 5 hrs 6 hrs 7 hrs 8 hrs 9 hrs 10 hrs

QUALITY OF SLEEP
☆ ☆ ☆ ☆ ☆

Describe your mood throughout the day. Note in particular the times when you felt 'high' or 'low'. What food/activity affected your mood and/or overall well-being today?

_____

_____

_____

_____

What did you crave today? When did you crave it, and why?
What did you do to manage your cravings throughout the day? Were you successful?

_____

_____

_____

_____

Additional notes/observations i.e. weight, muscle tone, shape, setbacks, motivation etc.

_____

_____

_____

_____

How can you make tomorrow even better?

_____

_____

_____

_____

DAY 4

M T W T F S S

DAY: _____   MONTH: _____   YEAR: _____

BREAKFAST	CALORIES	CARBS (g)	FAT (g)	PROTEIN (g)	FIBER (g)	SUGAR (g)	SODIUM (mg)
MORNING SNACK							
TOTAL:							

LUNCH	CALORIES	CARBS (g)	FAT (g)	PROTEIN (g)	FIBER (g)	SUGAR (g)	SODIUM (mg)
MIDDAY SNACK							
TOTAL:							

DINNER	CALORIES	CARBS (g)	FAT (g)	PROTEIN (g)	FIBER (g)	SUGAR (g)	SODIUM (mg)
EVENING SNACK							
TOTAL:							

DAILY TOTAL:

WATER INTAKE:

☐ ☐ ☐ ☐ ☐ ☐ ☐ ☐ ☐ ☐
1 OZ 2 OZ 3 OZ 4 OZ 5 OZ 6 OZ 7 OZ 8 OZ 9 OZ 10 OZ

TYPE OF EXERCISE/ACTIVITY	HOW LONG?	INTENSITY	CALORIES BURNED
	TOTAL CALORIES BURNED:		

SLEEP TRACKER:

○ ○ ○ ○ ○ ○ ○ ○ ○ ○
1 hr 2 hrs 3 hrs 4 hrs 5 hrs 6 hrs 7 hrs 8 hrs 9 hrs 10 hrs

QUALITY OF SLEEP
☆ ☆ ☆ ☆ ☆

Describe your mood throughout the day. Note in particular the times when you felt 'high' or 'low'. What food/activity affected your mood and/or overall well-being today?

_____

_____

_____

What did you crave today? When did you crave it, and why?
What did you do to manage your cravings throughout the day? Were you successful?

_____

_____

_____

Additional notes/observations i.e. weight, muscle tone, shape, setbacks, motivation etc.

_____

_____

_____

How can you make tomorrow even better?

_____

_____

_____

DAY 5

DAY: _____ MONTH: _____ YEAR: _____

BREAKFAST	CALORIES	CARBS (g)	FAT (g)	PROTEIN (g)	FIBER (g)	SUGAR (g)	SODIUM (mg)
MORNING SNACK							
TOTAL:							

LUNCH	CALORIES	CARBS (g)	FAT (g)	PROTEIN (g)	FIBER (g)	SUGAR (g)	SODIUM (mg)
MIDDAY SNACK							
TOTAL:							

DINNER	CALORIES	CARBS (g)	FAT (g)	PROTEIN (g)	FIBER (g)	SUGAR (g)	SODIUM (mg)
EVENING SNACK							
TOTAL:							

DAILY TOTAL:							

WATER INTAKE:

▢ ▢ ▢ ▢ ▢ ▢ ▢ ▢ ▢ ▢
1 OZ 2 OZ 3 OZ 4 OZ 5 OZ 6 OZ 7 OZ 8 OZ 9 OZ 10 OZ

TYPE OF EXERCISE/ACTIVITY	HOW LONG?	INTENSITY	CALORIES BURNED
	TOTAL CALORIES BURNED:		

SLEEP TRACKER:

○ ○ ○ ○ ○ ○ ○ ○ ○ ○
1 hr 2 hrs 3 hrs 4 hrs 5 hrs 6 hrs 7 hrs 8 hrs 9 hrs 10 hrs

QUALITY OF SLEEP
☆ ☆ ☆ ☆ ☆

Describe your mood throughout the day. Note in particular the times when you felt 'high' or 'low'. What food/activity affected your mood and/or overall well-being today?

_____

_____

_____

_____

What did you crave today? When did you crave it, and why?
What did you do to manage your cravings throughout the day? Were you successful?

_____

_____

_____

_____

Additional notes/observations i.e. weight, muscle tone, shape, setbacks, motivation etc.

_____

_____

_____

_____

How can you make tomorrow even better?

_____

_____

_____

_____

DAY 6

BREAKFAST	CALORIES	CARBS (g)	FAT (g)	PROTEIN (g)	FIBER (g)	SUGAR (g)	SODIUM (mg)
MORNING SNACK							
TOTAL:							

LUNCH	CALORIES	CARBS (g)	FAT (g)	PROTEIN (g)	FIBER (g)	SUGAR (g)	SODIUM (mg)
MIDDAY SNACK							
TOTAL:							

DINNER	CALORIES	CARBS (g)	FAT (g)	PROTEIN (g)	FIBER (g)	SUGAR (g)	SODIUM (mg)
EVENING SNACK							
TOTAL:							

DAILY TOTAL:							

WATER INTAKE:

☐ ☐ ☐ ☐ ☐ ☐ ☐ ☐ ☐ ☐

1 OZ   2 OZ   3 OZ   4 OZ   5 OZ   6 OZ   7 OZ   8 OZ   9 OZ   10 OZ

TYPE OF EXERCISE/ACTIVITY	HOW LONG?	INTENSITY	CALORIES BURNED
TOTAL CALORIES BURNED:			

SLEEP TRACKER:

◯ ◯ ◯ ◯ ◯ ◯ ◯ ◯ ◯ ◯
1 hr 2 hrs 3 hrs 4 hrs 5 hrs 6 hrs 7 hrs 8 hrs 9 hrs 10 hrs

QUALITY OF SLEEP
☆ ☆ ☆ ☆ ☆

Describe your mood throughout the day. Note in particular the times when you felt 'high' or 'low'. What food/activity affected your mood and/or overall well-being today?

_____

_____

_____

_____

What did you crave today? When did you crave it, and why?
What did you do to manage your cravings throughout the day? Were you successful?

_____

_____

_____

_____

Additional notes/observations i.e. weight, muscle tone, shape, setbacks, motivation etc.

_____

_____

_____

_____

How can you make tomorrow even better?

_____

_____

_____

_____

DAY 7

BREAKFAST	CALORIES	CARBS (g)	FAT (g)	PROTEIN (g)	FIBER (g)	SUGAR (g)	SODIUM (mg)
MORNING SNACK							
TOTAL:							

LUNCH	CALORIES	CARBS (g)	FAT (g)	PROTEIN (g)	FIBER (g)	SUGAR (g)	SODIUM (mg)
MIDDAY SNACK							
TOTAL:							

DINNER	CALORIES	CARBS (g)	FAT (g)	PROTEIN (g)	FIBER (g)	SUGAR (g)	SODIUM (mg)
EVENING SNACK							
TOTAL:							
DAILY TOTAL:							

WATER INTAKE:

☐   ☐   ☐   ☐   ☐   ☐   ☐   ☐   ☐   ☐
1 OZ   2 OZ   3 OZ   4 OZ   5 OZ   6 OZ   7 OZ   8 OZ   9 OZ   10 OZ

TYPE OF EXERCISE/ACTIVITY	HOW LONG?	INTENSITY	CALORIES BURNED
		TOTAL CALORIES BURNED:	

SLEEP TRACKER:

◯ ◯ ◯ ◯ ◯ ◯ ◯ ◯ ◯ ◯
1 hr 2 hrs 3 hrs 4 hrs 5 hrs 6 hrs 7 hrs 8 hrs 9 hrs 10 hrs

QUALITY OF SLEEP
☆ ☆ ☆ ☆ ☆

Describe your mood throughout the day. Note in particular the times when you felt 'high' or 'low'. What food/activity affected your mood and/or overall well-being today?

_____

_____

_____

_____

What did you crave today? When did you crave it, and why?
What did you do to manage your cravings throughout the day? Were you successful?

_____

_____

_____

_____

Additional notes/observations i.e. weight, muscle tone, shape, setbacks, motivation etc.

_____

_____

_____

_____

How can you make tomorrow even better?

_____

_____

_____

_____

DAY 8

BREAKFAST	CALORIES	CARBS (g)	FAT (g)	PROTEIN (g)	FIBER (g)	SUGAR (g)	SODIUM (mg)
MORNING SNACK							
TOTAL:							

LUNCH	CALORIES	CARBS (g)	FAT (g)	PROTEIN (g)	FIBER (g)	SUGAR (g)	SODIUM (mg)
MIDDAY SNACK							
TOTAL:							

DINNER	CALORIES	CARBS (g)	FAT (g)	PROTEIN (g)	FIBER (g)	SUGAR (g)	SODIUM (mg)
EVENING SNACK							
TOTAL:							

DAILY TOTAL:							

WATER INTAKE:

☐ ☐ ☐ ☐ ☐ ☐ ☐ ☐ ☐ ☐
1 OZ 2 OZ 3 OZ 4 OZ 5 OZ 6 OZ 7 OZ 8 OZ 9 OZ 10 OZ

TYPE OF EXERCISE/ACTIVITY	HOW LONG?	INTENSITY	CALORIES BURNED
TOTAL CALORIES BURNED:			

SLEEP TRACKER:

◯ ◯ ◯ ◯ ◯ ◯ ◯ ◯ ◯ ◯
1 hr   2 hrs   3 hrs   4 hrs   5 hrs   6 hrs   7 hrs   8 hrs   9 hrs   10 hrs

QUALITY OF SLEEP
☆ ☆ ☆ ☆ ☆

Describe your mood throughout the day. Note in particular the times when you felt 'high' or 'low'. What food/activity affected your mood and/or overall well-being today?

_____

_____

_____

_____

What did you crave today? When did you crave it, and why?
What did you do to manage your cravings throughout the day? Were you successful?

_____

_____

_____

_____

Additional notes/observations i.e. weight, muscle tone, shape, setbacks, motivation etc.

_____

_____

_____

_____

How can you make tomorrow even better?

_____

_____

_____

_____

DAY 9

BREAKFAST	CALORIES	CARBS (g)	FAT (g)	PROTEIN (g)	FIBER (g)	SUGAR (g)	SODIUM (mg)
MORNING SNACK							
TOTAL:							

LUNCH	CALORIES	CARBS (g)	FAT (g)	PROTEIN (g)	FIBER (g)	SUGAR (g)	SODIUM (mg)
MIDDAY SNACK							
TOTAL:							

DINNER	CALORIES	CARBS (g)	FAT (g)	PROTEIN (g)	FIBER (g)	SUGAR (g)	SODIUM (mg)
EVENING SNACK							
TOTAL:							

| DAILY TOTAL: | | | | | | | |

WATER INTAKE:

☐ ☐ ☐ ☐ ☐ ☐ ☐ ☐ ☐ ☐
1 OZ   2 OZ   3 OZ   4 OZ   5 OZ   6 OZ   7 OZ   8 OZ   9 OZ   10 OZ

TYPE OF EXERCISE/ACTIVITY	HOW LONG?	INTENSITY	CALORIES BURNED
	TOTAL CALORIES BURNED:		

SLEEP TRACKER:

○ ○ ○ ○ ○ ○ ○ ○ ○ ○
1 hr   2 hrs   3 hrs   4 hrs   5 hrs   6 hrs   7 hrs   8 hrs   9 hrs   10 hrs

QUALITY OF SLEEP
☆ ☆ ☆ ☆ ☆

Describe your mood throughout the day. Note in particular the times when you felt 'high' or 'low'. What food/activity affected your mood and/or overall well-being today?

_____

_____

_____

_____

What did you crave today? When did you crave it, and why?
What did you do to manage your cravings throughout the day? Were you successful?

_____

_____

_____

_____

Additional notes/observations i.e. weight, muscle tone, shape, setbacks, motivation etc.

_____

_____

_____

_____

How can you make tomorrow even better?

_____

_____

_____

DAY 10

BREAKFAST	CALORIES	CARBS (g)	FAT (g)	PROTEIN (g)	FIBER (g)	SUGAR (g)	SODIUM (mg)
MORNING SNACK							
TOTAL:							

LUNCH	CALORIES	CARBS (g)	FAT (g)	PROTEIN (g)	FIBER (g)	SUGAR (g)	SODIUM (mg)
MIDDAY SNACK							
TOTAL:							

DINNER	CALORIES	CARBS (g)	FAT (g)	PROTEIN (g)	FIBER (g)	SUGAR (g)	SODIUM (mg)
EVENING SNACK							
TOTAL:							

DAILY TOTAL:							

WATER INTAKE:

☐ ☐ ☐ ☐ ☐ ☐ ☐ ☐ ☐ ☐
1 OZ 2 OZ 3 OZ 4 OZ 5 OZ 6 OZ 7 OZ 8 OZ 9 OZ 10 OZ

TYPE OF EXERCISE/ACTIVITY	HOW LONG?	INTENSITY	CALORIES BURNED
	TOTAL CALORIES BURNED:		

SLEEP TRACKER:

○ ○ ○ ○ ○ ○ ○ ○ ○ ○
1 hr 2 hrs 3 hrs 4 hrs 5 hrs 6 hrs 7 hrs 8 hrs 9 hrs 10 hrs

QUALITY OF SLEEP
☆ ☆ ☆ ☆ ☆

Describe your mood throughout the day. Note in particular the times when you felt 'high' or 'low'. What food/activity affected your mood and/or overall well-being today?

_____

_____

_____

_____

What did you crave today? When did you crave it, and why?
What did you do to manage your cravings throughout the day? Were you successful?

_____

_____

_____

_____

Additional notes/observations i.e. weight, muscle tone, shape, setbacks, motivation etc.

_____

_____

_____

_____

How can you make tomorrow even better?

_____

_____

_____

_____

DAY 11

BREAKFAST	CALORIES	CARBS (g)	FAT (g)	PROTEIN (g)	FIBER (g)	SUGAR (g)	SODIUM (mg)
MORNING SNACK							
TOTAL:							

LUNCH	CALORIES	CARBS (g)	FAT (g)	PROTEIN (g)	FIBER (g)	SUGAR (g)	SODIUM (mg)
MIDDAY SNACK							
TOTAL:							

DINNER	CALORIES	CARBS (g)	FAT (g)	PROTEIN (g)	FIBER (g)	SUGAR (g)	SODIUM (mg)
EVENING SNACK							
TOTAL:							

DAILY TOTAL:							

WATER INTAKE:

☐ ☐ ☐ ☐ ☐ ☐ ☐ ☐ ☐ ☐
1 OZ 2 OZ 3 OZ 4 OZ 5 OZ 6 OZ 7 OZ 8 OZ 9 OZ 10 OZ

TYPE OF EXERCISE/ACTIVITY	HOW LONG?	INTENSITY	CALORIES BURNED
	TOTAL CALORIES BURNED:		

SLEEP TRACKER:

◯   ◯   ◯   ◯   ◯   ◯   ◯   ◯   ◯   ◯

1 hr   2 hrs   3 hrs   4 hrs   5 hrs   6 hrs   7 hrs   8 hrs   9 hrs   10 hrs

QUALITY OF SLEEP

☆ ☆ ☆ ☆ ☆

Describe your mood throughout the day. Note in particular the times when you felt 'high' or 'low'. What food/activity affected your mood and/or overall well-being today?

_____

_____

_____

_____

What did you crave today? When did you crave it, and why?
What did you do to manage your cravings throughout the day? Were you successful?

_____

_____

_____

_____

Additional notes/observations i.e. weight, muscle tone, shape, setbacks, motivation etc.

_____

_____

_____

_____

How can you make tomorrow even better?

_____

_____

_____

_____

DAY 12

BREAKFAST	CALORIES	CARBS (g)	FAT (g)	PROTEIN (g)	FIBER (g)	SUGAR (g)	SODIUM (mg)
MORNING SNACK							
TOTAL:							

LUNCH	CALORIES	CARBS (g)	FAT (g)	PROTEIN (g)	FIBER (g)	SUGAR (g)	SODIUM (mg)
MIDDAY SNACK							
TOTAL:							

DINNER	CALORIES	CARBS (g)	FAT (g)	PROTEIN (g)	FIBER (g)	SUGAR (g)	SODIUM (mg)
EVENING SNACK							
TOTAL:							
DAILY TOTAL:							

WATER INTAKE:

☐ ☐ ☐ ☐ ☐ ☐ ☐ ☐ ☐ ☐
1 OZ   2 OZ   3 OZ   4 OZ   5 OZ   6 OZ   7 OZ   8 OZ   9 OZ   10 OZ

TYPE OF EXERCISE/ACTIVITY	HOW LONG?	INTENSITY	CALORIES BURNED
TOTAL CALORIES BURNED:			

SLEEP TRACKER:

○   ○   ○   ○   ○   ○   ○   ○   ○   ○
1 hr   2 hrs   3 hrs   4 hrs   5 hrs   6 hrs   7 hrs   8 hrs   9 hrs   10 hrs

QUALITY OF SLEEP
☆ ☆ ☆ ☆ ☆

Describe your mood throughout the day. Note in particular the times when you felt 'high' or 'low'. What food/activity affected your mood and/or overall well-being today?

_____

_____

_____

_____

What did you crave today? When did you crave it, and why?
What did you do to manage your cravings throughout the day? Were you successful?

_____

_____

_____

_____

Additional notes/observations i.e. weight, muscle tone, shape, setbacks, motivation etc.

_____

_____

_____

_____

How can you make tomorrow even better?

_____

_____

_____

_____

DAY 13

BREAKFAST	CALORIES	CARBS (g)	FAT (g)	PROTEIN (g)	FIBER (g)	SUGAR (g)	SODIUM (mg)
MORNING SNACK							
TOTAL:							

LUNCH	CALORIES	CARBS (g)	FAT (g)	PROTEIN (g)	FIBER (g)	SUGAR (g)	SODIUM (mg)
MIDDAY SNACK							
TOTAL:							

DINNER	CALORIES	CARBS (g)	FAT (g)	PROTEIN (g)	FIBER (g)	SUGAR (g)	SODIUM (mg)
EVENING SNACK							
TOTAL:							
DAILY TOTAL:							

WATER INTAKE:

☐ ☐ ☐ ☐ ☐ ☐ ☐ ☐ ☐ ☐
1 OZ 2 OZ 3 OZ 4 OZ 5 OZ 6 OZ 7 OZ 8 OZ 9 OZ 10 OZ

TYPE OF EXERCISE/ACTIVITY	HOW LONG?	INTENSITY	CALORIES BURNED
		TOTAL CALORIES BURNED:	

SLEEP TRACKER:

○ ○ ○ ○ ○ ○ ○ ○ ○ ○
1 hr 2 hrs 3 hrs 4 hrs 5 hrs 6 hrs 7 hrs 8 hrs 9 hrs 10 hrs

QUALITY OF SLEEP
☆ ☆ ☆ ☆ ☆

Describe your mood throughout the day. Note in particular the times when you felt 'high' or 'low'. What food/activity affected your mood and/or overall well-being today?

_____

_____

_____

_____

What did you crave today? When did you crave it, and why?
What did you do to manage your cravings throughout the day? Were you successful?

_____

_____

_____

_____

Additional notes/observations i.e. weight, muscle tone, shape, setbacks, motivation etc.

_____

_____

_____

_____

How can you make tomorrow even better?

_____

_____

_____

_____

DAY 14

BREAKFAST	CALORIES	CARBS (g)	FAT (g)	PROTEIN (g)	FIBER (g)	SUGAR (g)	SODIUM (mg)
MORNING SNACK							
TOTAL:							

LUNCH	CALORIES	CARBS (g)	FAT (g)	PROTEIN (g)	FIBER (g)	SUGAR (g)	SODIUM (mg)
MIDDAY SNACK							
TOTAL:							

DINNER	CALORIES	CARBS (g)	FAT (g)	PROTEIN (g)	FIBER (g)	SUGAR (g)	SODIUM (mg)
EVENING SNACK							
TOTAL:							

DAILY TOTAL:							

WATER INTAKE:

☐ ☐ ☐ ☐ ☐ ☐ ☐ ☐ ☐ ☐
1 OZ 2 OZ 3 OZ 4 OZ 5 OZ 6 OZ 7 OZ 8 OZ 9 OZ 10 OZ

TYPE OF EXERCISE/ACTIVITY	HOW LONG?	INTENSITY	CALORIES BURNED
		TOTAL CALORIES BURNED:	

SLEEP TRACKER:

○ ○ ○ ○ ○ ○ ○ ○ ○ ○
1 hr 2 hrs 3 hrs 4 hrs 5 hrs 6 hrs 7 hrs 8 hrs 9 hrs 10 hrs

QUALITY OF SLEEP
☆ ☆ ☆ ☆ ☆

Describe your mood throughout the day. Note in particular the times when you felt 'high' or 'low'. What food/activity affected your mood and/or overall well-being today?

_____

_____

_____

_____

What did you crave today? When did you crave it, and why?
What did you do to manage your cravings throughout the day? Were you successful?

_____

_____

_____

_____

Additional notes/observations i.e. weight, muscle tone, shape, setbacks, motivation etc.

_____

_____

_____

_____

How can you make tomorrow even better?

_____

_____

_____

_____

DAY 15

BREAKFAST	CALORIES	CARBS (g)	FAT (g)	PROTEIN (g)	FIBER (g)	SUGAR (g)	SODIUM (mg)
MORNING SNACK							
TOTAL:							

LUNCH	CALORIES	CARBS (g)	FAT (g)	PROTEIN (g)	FIBER (g)	SUGAR (g)	SODIUM (mg)
MIDDAY SNACK							
TOTAL:							

DINNER	CALORIES	CARBS (g)	FAT (g)	PROTEIN (g)	FIBER (g)	SUGAR (g)	SODIUM (mg)
EVENING SNACK							
TOTAL:							
DAILY TOTAL:							

WATER INTAKE:

☐ ☐ ☐ ☐ ☐ ☐ ☐ ☐ ☐ ☐
1 OZ 2 OZ 3 OZ 4 OZ 5 OZ 6 OZ 7 OZ 8 OZ 9 OZ 10 OZ

TYPE OF EXERCISE/ACTIVITY	HOW LONG?	INTENSITY	CALORIES BURNED
TOTAL CALORIES BURNED:			

SLEEP TRACKER:

◯ ◯ ◯ ◯ ◯ ◯ ◯ ◯ ◯ ◯
1 hr 2 hrs 3 hrs 4 hrs 5 hrs 6 hrs 7 hrs 8 hrs 9 hrs 10 hrs

QUALITY OF SLEEP
☆ ☆ ☆ ☆ ☆

Describe your mood throughout the day. Note in particular the times when you felt 'high' or 'low'. What food/activity affected your mood and/or overall well-being today?

_____

_____

_____

_____

What did you crave today? When did you crave it, and why?
What did you do to manage your cravings throughout the day? Were you successful?

_____

_____

_____

_____

Additional notes/observations i.e. weight, muscle tone, shape, setbacks, motivation etc.

_____

_____

_____

_____

How can you make tomorrow even better?

_____

_____

_____

_____

DAY 16

M T W T F S S

DAY: _____   MONTH: _____   YEAR: _____

BREAKFAST	CALORIES	CARBS (g)	FAT (g)	PROTEIN (g)	FIBER (g)	SUGAR (g)	SODIUM (mg)
MORNING SNACK							
TOTAL:							

LUNCH	CALORIES	CARBS (g)	FAT (g)	PROTEIN (g)	FIBER (g)	SUGAR (g)	SODIUM (mg)
MIDDAY SNACK							
TOTAL:							

DINNER	CALORIES	CARBS (g)	FAT (g)	PROTEIN (g)	FIBER (g)	SUGAR (g)	SODIUM (mg)
EVENING SNACK							
TOTAL:							

DAILY TOTAL:							

WATER INTAKE:

☐ ☐ ☐ ☐ ☐ ☐ ☐ ☐ ☐ ☐
1 OZ 2 OZ 3 OZ 4 OZ 5 OZ 6 OZ 7 OZ 8 OZ 9 OZ 10 OZ

TYPE OF EXERCISE/ACTIVITY	HOW LONG?	INTENSITY	CALORIES BURNED
TOTAL CALORIES BURNED:			

SLEEP TRACKER:

○   ○   ○   ○   ○   ○   ○   ○   ○   ○

1 hr   2 hrs   3 hrs   4 hrs   5 hrs   6 hrs   7 hrs   8 hrs   9 hrs   10 hrs

QUALITY OF SLEEP

☆ ☆ ☆ ☆ ☆

Describe your mood throughout the day. Note in particular the times when you felt 'high' or 'low'. What food/activity affected your mood and/or overall well-being today?

_____

_____

_____

_____

What did you crave today? When did you crave it, and why?
What did you do to manage your cravings throughout the day? Were you successful?

_____

_____

_____

_____

Additional notes/observations i.e. weight, muscle tone, shape, setbacks, motivation etc.

_____

_____

_____

_____

How can you make tomorrow even better?

_____

_____

_____

_____

DAY 17

M　T　W　T　F　S　S

DAY: _____　MONTH: _____　YEAR: _____

BREAKFAST	CALORIES	CARBS (g)	FAT (g)	PROTEIN (g)	FIBER (g)	SUGAR (g)	SODIUM (mg)
MORNING SNACK							
TOTAL:							

LUNCH	CALORIES	CARBS (g)	FAT (g)	PROTEIN (g)	FIBER (g)	SUGAR (g)	SODIUM (mg)
MIDDAY SNACK							
TOTAL:							

DINNER	CALORIES	CARBS (g)	FAT (g)	PROTEIN (g)	FIBER (g)	SUGAR (g)	SODIUM (mg)
EVENING SNACK							
TOTAL:							

DAILY TOTAL:

WATER INTAKE:

☐　☐　☐　☐　☐　☐　☐　☐　☐　☐
1 OZ　2 OZ　3 OZ　4 OZ　5 OZ　6 OZ　7 OZ　8 OZ　9 OZ　10 OZ

TYPE OF EXERCISE/ACTIVITY	HOW LONG?	INTENSITY	CALORIES BURNED
TOTAL CALORIES BURNED:			

SLEEP TRACKER:

○ ○ ○ ○ ○ ○ ○ ○ ○ ○
1 hr 2 hrs 3 hrs 4 hrs 5 hrs 6 hrs 7 hrs 8 hrs 9 hrs 10 hrs

QUALITY OF SLEEP
☆ ☆ ☆ ☆ ☆

Describe your mood throughout the day. Note in particular the times when you felt 'high' or 'low'. What food/activity affected your mood and/or overall well-being today?

_____

_____

_____

_____

What did you crave today? When did you crave it, and why?
What did you do to manage your cravings throughout the day? Were you successful?

_____

_____

_____

_____

Additional notes/observations i.e. weight, muscle tone, shape, setbacks, motivation etc.

_____

_____

_____

_____

How can you make tomorrow even better?

_____

_____

_____

DAY 18

DAY: _____   MONTH: _____   YEAR: _____

BREAKFAST	CALORIES	CARBS (g)	FAT (g)	PROTEIN (g)	FIBER (g)	SUGAR (g)	SODIUM (mg)
MORNING SNACK							
TOTAL:							

LUNCH	CALORIES	CARBS (g)	FAT (g)	PROTEIN (g)	FIBER (g)	SUGAR (g)	SODIUM (mg)
MIDDAY SNACK							
TOTAL:							

DINNER	CALORIES	CARBS (g)	FAT (g)	PROTEIN (g)	FIBER (g)	SUGAR (g)	SODIUM (mg)
EVENING SNACK							
TOTAL:							

DAILY TOTAL:							

WATER INTAKE:

☐ ☐ ☐ ☐ ☐ ☐ ☐ ☐ ☐ ☐
1 OZ 2 OZ 3 OZ 4 OZ 5 OZ 6 OZ 7 OZ 8 OZ 9 OZ 10 OZ

TYPE OF EXERCISE/ACTIVITY	HOW LONG?	INTENSITY	CALORIES BURNED
		TOTAL CALORIES BURNED:	

SLEEP TRACKER:

○ ○ ○ ○ ○ ○ ○ ○ ○ ○
1 hr 2 hrs 3 hrs 4 hrs 5 hrs 6 hrs 7 hrs 8 hrs 9 hrs 10 hrs

QUALITY OF SLEEP
☆ ☆ ☆ ☆ ☆

Describe your mood throughout the day. Note in particular the times when you felt 'high' or 'low'. What food/activity affected your mood and/or overall well-being today?

_____

_____

_____

_____

What did you crave today? When did you crave it, and why?
What did you do to manage your cravings throughout the day? Were you successful?

_____

_____

_____

_____

Additional notes/observations i.e. weight, muscle tone, shape, setbacks, motivation etc.

_____

_____

_____

_____

How can you make tomorrow even better?

_____

_____

_____

_____

DAY 19

BREAKFAST	CALORIES	CARBS (g)	FAT (g)	PROTEIN (g)	FIBER (g)	SUGAR (g)	SODIUM (mg)
MORNING SNACK							
TOTAL:							

LUNCH	CALORIES	CARBS (g)	FAT (g)	PROTEIN (g)	FIBER (g)	SUGAR (g)	SODIUM (mg)
MIDDAY SNACK							
TOTAL:							

DINNER	CALORIES	CARBS (g)	FAT (g)	PROTEIN (g)	FIBER (g)	SUGAR (g)	SODIUM (mg)
EVENING SNACK							
TOTAL:							

| DAILY TOTAL: | | | | | | | |

WATER INTAKE:

☐ 1 OZ ☐ 2 OZ ☐ 3 OZ ☐ 4 OZ ☐ 5 OZ ☐ 6 OZ ☐ 7 OZ ☐ 8 OZ ☐ 9 OZ ☐ 10 OZ

TYPE OF EXERCISE/ACTIVITY	HOW LONG?	INTENSITY	CALORIES BURNED
		TOTAL CALORIES BURNED:	

SLEEP TRACKER:

○   ○   ○   ○   ○   ○   ○   ○   ○   ○

1 hr   2 hrs   3 hrs   4 hrs   5 hrs   6 hrs   7 hrs   8 hrs   9 hrs   10 hrs

QUALITY OF SLEEP

☆ ☆ ☆ ☆ ☆

Describe your mood throughout the day. Note in particular the times when you felt 'high' or 'low'. What food/activity affected your mood and/or overall well-being today?

_____

_____

_____

_____

What did you crave today? When did you crave it, and why?
What did you do to manage your cravings throughout the day? Were you successful?

_____

_____

_____

_____

Additional notes/observations i.e. weight, muscle tone, shape, setbacks, motivation etc.

_____

_____

_____

_____

How can you make tomorrow even better?

_____

_____

_____

_____

DAY 20

BREAKFAST	CALORIES	CARBS (g)	FAT (g)	PROTEIN (g)	FIBER (g)	SUGAR (g)	SODIUM (mg)
MORNING SNACK							
TOTAL:							

LUNCH	CALORIES	CARBS (g)	FAT (g)	PROTEIN (g)	FIBER (g)	SUGAR (g)	SODIUM (mg)
MIDDAY SNACK							
TOTAL:							

DINNER	CALORIES	CARBS (g)	FAT (g)	PROTEIN (g)	FIBER (g)	SUGAR (g)	SODIUM (mg)
EVENING SNACK							
TOTAL:							

DAILY TOTAL:

WATER INTAKE:

☐ ☐ ☐ ☐ ☐ ☐ ☐ ☐ ☐ ☐
1 OZ 2 OZ 3 OZ 4 OZ 5 OZ 6 OZ 7 OZ 8 OZ 9 OZ 10 OZ

TYPE OF EXERCISE/ACTIVITY	HOW LONG?	INTENSITY	CALORIES BURNED
		TOTAL CALORIES BURNED:	

SLEEP TRACKER:

○ ○ ○ ○ ○ ○ ○ ○ ○ ○
1 hr   2 hrs   3 hrs   4 hrs   5 hrs   6 hrs   7 hrs   8 hrs   9 hrs   10 hrs

QUALITY OF SLEEP
☆ ☆ ☆ ☆ ☆

Describe your mood throughout the day. Note in particular the times when you felt 'high' or 'low'. What food/activity affected your mood and/or overall well-being today?

_____

_____

_____

What did you crave today? When did you crave it, and why?
What did you do to manage your cravings throughout the day? Were you successful?

_____

_____

_____

Additional notes/observations i.e. weight, muscle tone, shape, setbacks, motivation etc.

_____

_____

_____

How can you make tomorrow even better?

_____

_____

_____

DAY 21

BREAKFAST	CALORIES	CARBS (g)	FAT (g)	PROTEIN (g)	FIBER (g)	SUGAR (g)	SODIUM (mg)
MORNING SNACK							
TOTAL:							

LUNCH	CALORIES	CARBS (g)	FAT (g)	PROTEIN (g)	FIBER (g)	SUGAR (g)	SODIUM (mg)
MIDDAY SNACK							
TOTAL:							

DINNER	CALORIES	CARBS (g)	FAT (g)	PROTEIN (g)	FIBER (g)	SUGAR (g)	SODIUM (mg)
EVENING SNACK							
TOTAL:							
DAILY TOTAL:							

WATER INTAKE:

☐ ☐ ☐ ☐ ☐ ☐ ☐ ☐ ☐ ☐
1 OZ   2 OZ   3 OZ   4 OZ   5 OZ   6 OZ   7 OZ   8 OZ   9 OZ   10 OZ

TYPE OF EXERCISE/ACTIVITY	HOW LONG?	INTENSITY	CALORIES BURNED
	TOTAL CALORIES BURNED:		

SLEEP TRACKER:

○ ○ ○ ○ ○ ○ ○ ○ ○ ○
1 hr 2 hrs 3 hrs 4 hrs 5 hrs 6 hrs 7 hrs 8 hrs 9 hrs 10 hrs

QUALITY OF SLEEP
☆ ☆ ☆ ☆ ☆

Describe your mood throughout the day. Note in particular the times when you felt 'high' or 'low'. What food/activity affected your mood and/or overall well-being today?

_____

_____

_____

_____

What did you crave today? When did you crave it, and why?
What did you do to manage your cravings throughout the day? Were you successful?

_____

_____

_____

_____

Additional notes/observations i.e. weight, muscle tone, shape, setbacks, motivation etc.

_____

_____

_____

_____

How can you make tomorrow even better?

_____

_____

_____

DAY 22

BREAKFAST	CALORIES	CARBS (g)	FAT (g)	PROTEIN (g)	FIBER (g)	SUGAR (g)	SODIUM (mg)
MORNING SNACK							
TOTAL:							

LUNCH	CALORIES	CARBS (g)	FAT (g)	PROTEIN (g)	FIBER (g)	SUGAR (g)	SODIUM (mg)
MIDDAY SNACK							
TOTAL:							

DINNER	CALORIES	CARBS (g)	FAT (g)	PROTEIN (g)	FIBER (g)	SUGAR (g)	SODIUM (mg)
EVENING SNACK							
TOTAL:							
DAILY TOTAL:							

WATER INTAKE:

☐   ☐   ☐   ☐   ☐   ☐   ☐   ☐   ☐   ☐
1 OZ   2 OZ   3 OZ   4 OZ   5 OZ   6 OZ   7 OZ   8 OZ   9 OZ   10 OZ

TYPE OF EXERCISE/ACTIVITY	HOW LONG?	INTENSITY	CALORIES BURNED
		TOTAL CALORIES BURNED:	

SLEEP TRACKER:

○ ○ ○ ○ ○ ○ ○ ○ ○ ○
1 hr 2 hrs 3 hrs 4 hrs 5 hrs 6 hrs 7 hrs 8 hrs 9 hrs 10 hrs

QUALITY OF SLEEP
☆ ☆ ☆ ☆ ☆

Describe your mood throughout the day. Note in particular the times when you felt 'high' or 'low'. What food/activity affected your mood and/or overall well-being today?

_____

_____

_____

_____

What did you crave today? When did you crave it, and why?
What did you do to manage your cravings throughout the day? Were you successful?

_____

_____

_____

_____

Additional notes/observations i.e. weight, muscle tone, shape, setbacks, motivation etc.

_____

_____

_____

_____

How can you make tomorrow even better?

_____

_____

_____

_____

DAY 23

BREAKFAST	CALORIES	CARBS (g)	FAT (g)	PROTEIN (g)	FIBER (g)	SUGAR (g)	SODIUM (mg)
MORNING SNACK							
TOTAL:							

LUNCH	CALORIES	CARBS (g)	FAT (g)	PROTEIN (g)	FIBER (g)	SUGAR (g)	SODIUM (mg)
MIDDAY SNACK							
TOTAL:							

DINNER	CALORIES	CARBS (g)	FAT (g)	PROTEIN (g)	FIBER (g)	SUGAR (g)	SODIUM (mg)
EVENING SNACK							
TOTAL:							

DAILY TOTAL:							

WATER INTAKE:

☐ ☐ ☐ ☐ ☐ ☐ ☐ ☐ ☐ ☐
1 OZ 2 OZ 3 OZ 4 OZ 5 OZ 6 OZ 7 OZ 8 OZ 9 OZ 10 OZ

TYPE OF EXERCISE/ACTIVITY	HOW LONG?	INTENSITY	CALORIES BURNED
TOTAL CALORIES BURNED:			

SLEEP TRACKER:

○ ○ ○ ○ ○ ○ ○ ○ ○ ○
1 hr 2 hrs 3 hrs 4 hrs 5 hrs 6 hrs 7 hrs 8 hrs 9 hrs 10 hrs

QUALITY OF SLEEP
☆ ☆ ☆ ☆ ☆

Describe your mood throughout the day. Note in particular the times when you felt 'high' or 'low'. What food/activity affected your mood and/or overall well-being today?

_____

_____

_____

_____

What did you crave today? When did you crave it, and why?
What did you do to manage your cravings throughout the day? Were you successful?

_____

_____

_____

_____

Additional notes/observations i.e. weight, muscle tone, shape, setbacks, motivation etc.

_____

_____

_____

_____

How can you make tomorrow even better?

_____

_____

_____

_____

DAY 24

DAY: _____   MONTH: _____   YEAR: _____

BREAKFAST	CALORIES	CARBS (g)	FAT (g)	PROTEIN (g)	FIBER (g)	SUGAR (g)	SODIUM (mg)
MORNING SNACK							
TOTAL:							

LUNCH	CALORIES	CARBS (g)	FAT (g)	PROTEIN (g)	FIBER (g)	SUGAR (g)	SODIUM (mg)
MIDDAY SNACK							
TOTAL:							

DINNER	CALORIES	CARBS (g)	FAT (g)	PROTEIN (g)	FIBER (g)	SUGAR (g)	SODIUM (mg)
EVENING SNACK							
TOTAL:							

DAILY TOTAL:							

WATER INTAKE:

☐ ☐ ☐ ☐ ☐ ☐ ☐ ☐ ☐ ☐
1 OZ   2 OZ   3 OZ   4 OZ   5 OZ   6 OZ   7 OZ   8 OZ   9 OZ   10 OZ

TYPE OF EXERCISE/ACTIVITY	HOW LONG?	INTENSITY	CALORIES BURNED
TOTAL CALORIES BURNED:			

SLEEP TRACKER:

○   ○   ○   ○   ○   ○   ○   ○   ○   ○

1 hr   2 hrs   3 hrs   4 hrs   5 hrs   6 hrs   7 hrs   8 hrs   9 hrs   10 hrs

QUALITY OF SLEEP

☆ ☆ ☆ ☆ ☆

Describe your mood throughout the day. Note in particular the times when you felt 'high' or 'low'. What food/activity affected your mood and/or overall well-being today?

_____

_____

_____

_____

What did you crave today? When did you crave it, and why?
What did you do to manage your cravings throughout the day? Were you successful?

_____

_____

_____

_____

Additional notes/observations i.e. weight, muscle tone, shape, setbacks, motivation etc.

_____

_____

_____

_____

How can you make tomorrow even better?

_____

_____

_____

_____

DAY 25

DAY: _____ MONTH: _____ YEAR: _____

BREAKFAST	CALORIES	CARBS (g)	FAT (g)	PROTEIN (g)	FIBER (g)	SUGAR (g)	SODIUM (mg)
MORNING SNACK							
TOTAL:							

LUNCH	CALORIES	CARBS (g)	FAT (g)	PROTEIN (g)	FIBER (g)	SUGAR (g)	SODIUM (mg)
MIDDAY SNACK							
TOTAL:							

DINNER	CALORIES	CARBS (g)	FAT (g)	PROTEIN (g)	FIBER (g)	SUGAR (g)	SODIUM (mg)
EVENING SNACK							
TOTAL:							

DAILY TOTAL:

WATER INTAKE:

☐ ☐ ☐ ☐ ☐ ☐ ☐ ☐ ☐ ☐
1 OZ 2 OZ 3 OZ 4 OZ 5 OZ 6 OZ 7 OZ 8 OZ 9 OZ 10 OZ

TYPE OF EXERCISE/ACTIVITY	HOW LONG?	INTENSITY	CALORIES BURNED
TOTAL CALORIES BURNED:			

SLEEP TRACKER:

○ ○ ○ ○ ○ ○ ○ ○ ○ ○
1 hr 2 hrs 3 hrs 4 hrs 5 hrs 6 hrs 7 hrs 8 hrs 9 hrs 10 hrs

QUALITY OF SLEEP
☆ ☆ ☆ ☆ ☆

Describe your mood throughout the day. Note in particular the times when you felt 'high' or 'low'. What food/activity affected your mood and/or overall well-being today?

_____

_____

_____

_____

What did you crave today? When did you crave it, and why?
What did you do to manage your cravings throughout the day? Were you successful?

_____

_____

_____

_____

Additional notes/observations i.e. weight, muscle tone, shape, setbacks, motivation etc.

_____

_____

_____

_____

How can you make tomorrow even better?

_____

_____

_____

_____

DAY 26

DAY: _____   MONTH: _____   YEAR: _____

BREAKFAST	CALORIES	CARBS (g)	FAT (g)	PROTEIN (g)	FIBER (g)	SUGAR (g)	SODIUM (mg)
MORNING SNACK							
TOTAL:							

LUNCH	CALORIES	CARBS (g)	FAT (g)	PROTEIN (g)	FIBER (g)	SUGAR (g)	SODIUM (mg)
MIDDAY SNACK							
TOTAL:							

DINNER	CALORIES	CARBS (g)	FAT (g)	PROTEIN (g)	FIBER (g)	SUGAR (g)	SODIUM (mg)
EVENING SNACK							
TOTAL:							

| DAILY TOTAL: | | | | | | | |

WATER INTAKE:

☐ ☐ ☐ ☐ ☐ ☐ ☐ ☐ ☐ ☐
1 OZ 2 OZ 3 OZ 4 OZ 5 OZ 6 OZ 7 OZ 8 OZ 9 OZ 10 OZ

TYPE OF EXERCISE/ACTIVITY	HOW LONG?	INTENSITY	CALORIES BURNED
		TOTAL CALORIES BURNED:	

SLEEP TRACKER:

◯   ◯   ◯   ◯   ◯   ◯   ◯   ◯   ◯   ◯

1 hr   2 hrs   3 hrs   4 hrs   5 hrs   6 hrs   7 hrs   8 hrs   9 hrs   10 hrs

QUALITY OF SLEEP

☆ ☆ ☆ ☆ ☆

Describe your mood throughout the day. Note in particular the times when you felt 'high' or 'low'. What food/activity affected your mood and/or overall well-being today?

_____

_____

_____

_____

What did you crave today? When did you crave it, and why?
What did you do to manage your cravings throughout the day? Were you successful?

_____

_____

_____

_____

Additional notes/observations i.e. weight, muscle tone, shape, setbacks, motivation etc.

_____

_____

_____

_____

How can you make tomorrow even better?

_____

_____

_____

_____

DAY 27

BREAKFAST	CALORIES	CARBS (g)	FAT (g)	PROTEIN (g)	FIBER (g)	SUGAR (g)	SODIUM (mg)
MORNING SNACK							
TOTAL:							

LUNCH	CALORIES	CARBS (g)	FAT (g)	PROTEIN (g)	FIBER (g)	SUGAR (g)	SODIUM (mg)
MIDDAY SNACK							
TOTAL:							

DINNER	CALORIES	CARBS (g)	FAT (g)	PROTEIN (g)	FIBER (g)	SUGAR (g)	SODIUM (mg)
EVENING SNACK							
TOTAL:							

| DAILY TOTAL: | | | | | | | |

WATER INTAKE:

1 OZ   2 OZ   3 OZ   4 OZ   5 OZ   6 OZ   7 OZ   8 OZ   9 OZ   10 OZ

TYPE OF EXERCISE/ACTIVITY	HOW LONG?	INTENSITY	CALORIES BURNED
		TOTAL CALORIES BURNED:	

SLEEP TRACKER:

○ ○ ○ ○ ○ ○ ○ ○ ○ ○
1 hr   2 hrs   3 hrs   4 hrs   5 hrs   6 hrs   7 hrs   8 hrs   9 hrs   10 hrs

QUALITY OF SLEEP
☆ ☆ ☆ ☆ ☆

Describe your mood throughout the day. Note in particular the times when you felt 'high' or 'low'. What food/activity affected your mood and/or overall well-being today?

_____

_____

_____

_____

What did you crave today? When did you crave it, and why?
What did you do to manage your cravings throughout the day? Were you successful?

_____

_____

_____

_____

Additional notes/observations i.e. weight, muscle tone, shape, setbacks, motivation etc.

_____

_____

_____

_____

How can you make tomorrow even better?

_____

_____

_____

_____

DAY 28

M T W T F S S

DAY: _____ MONTH: _____ YEAR: _____

BREAKFAST	CALORIES	CARBS (g)	FAT (g)	PROTEIN (g)	FIBER (g)	SUGAR (g)	SODIUM (mg)
MORNING SNACK							
TOTAL:							

LUNCH	CALORIES	CARBS (g)	FAT (g)	PROTEIN (g)	FIBER (g)	SUGAR (g)	SODIUM (mg)
MIDDAY SNACK							
TOTAL:							

DINNER	CALORIES	CARBS (g)	FAT (g)	PROTEIN (g)	FIBER (g)	SUGAR (g)	SODIUM (mg)
EVENING SNACK							
TOTAL:							

DAILY TOTAL:							

WATER INTAKE:

☐ ☐ ☐ ☐ ☐ ☐ ☐ ☐ ☐ ☐
1 OZ 2 OZ 3 OZ 4 OZ 5 OZ 6 OZ 7 OZ 8 OZ 9 OZ 10 OZ

TYPE OF EXERCISE/ACTIVITY	HOW LONG?	INTENSITY	CALORIES BURNED
TOTAL CALORIES BURNED:			

SLEEP TRACKER:

○ ○ ○ ○ ○ ○ ○ ○ ○ ○
1 hr 2 hrs 3 hrs 4 hrs 5 hrs 6 hrs 7 hrs 8 hrs 9 hrs 10 hrs

QUALITY OF SLEEP
☆ ☆ ☆ ☆ ☆

Describe your mood throughout the day. Note in particular the times when you felt 'high' or 'low'. What food/activity affected your mood and/or overall well-being today?

_____

_____

_____

_____

What did you crave today? When did you crave it, and why?
What did you do to manage your cravings throughout the day? Were you successful?

_____

_____

_____

_____

Additional notes/observations i.e. weight, muscle tone, shape, setbacks, motivation etc.

_____

_____

_____

_____

How can you make tomorrow even better?

_____

_____

_____

_____

DAY 29

BREAKFAST	CALORIES	CARBS (g)	FAT (g)	PROTEIN (g)	FIBER (g)	SUGAR (g)	SODIUM (mg)
MORNING SNACK							
TOTAL:							

LUNCH	CALORIES	CARBS (g)	FAT (g)	PROTEIN (g)	FIBER (g)	SUGAR (g)	SODIUM (mg)
MIDDAY SNACK							
TOTAL:							

DINNER	CALORIES	CARBS (g)	FAT (g)	PROTEIN (g)	FIBER (g)	SUGAR (g)	SODIUM (mg)
EVENING SNACK							
TOTAL:							
DAILY TOTAL:							

WATER INTAKE:

▢ ▢ ▢ ▢ ▢ ▢ ▢ ▢ ▢ ▢
1 OZ 2 OZ 3 OZ 4 OZ 5 OZ 6 OZ 7 OZ 8 OZ 9 OZ 10 OZ

TYPE OF EXERCISE/ACTIVITY	HOW LONG?	INTENSITY	CALORIES BURNED
		TOTAL CALORIES BURNED:	

SLEEP TRACKER:

○ ○ ○ ○ ○ ○ ○ ○ ○ ○
1 hr 2 hrs 3 hrs 4 hrs 5 hrs 6 hrs 7 hrs 8 hrs 9 hrs 10 hrs

QUALITY OF SLEEP
☆ ☆ ☆ ☆ ☆

Describe your mood throughout the day. Note in particular the times when you felt 'high' or 'low'. What food/activity affected your mood and/or overall well-being today?

_____

_____

_____

_____

What did you crave today? When did you crave it, and why?
What did you do to manage your cravings throughout the day? Were you successful?

_____

_____

_____

Additional notes/observations i.e. weight, muscle tone, shape, setbacks, motivation etc.

_____

_____

_____

_____

How can you make tomorrow even better?

_____

_____

_____

_____

DAY 30

BREAKFAST	CALORIES	CARBS (g)	FAT (g)	PROTEIN (g)	FIBER (g)	SUGAR (g)	SODIUM (mg)
MORNING SNACK							
TOTAL:							

LUNCH	CALORIES	CARBS (g)	FAT (g)	PROTEIN (g)	FIBER (g)	SUGAR (g)	SODIUM (mg)
MIDDAY SNACK							
TOTAL:							

DINNER	CALORIES	CARBS (g)	FAT (g)	PROTEIN (g)	FIBER (g)	SUGAR (g)	SODIUM (mg)
EVENING SNACK							
TOTAL:							
DAILY TOTAL:							

WATER INTAKE:

☐ ☐ ☐ ☐ ☐ ☐ ☐ ☐ ☐ ☐
1 OZ   2 OZ   3 OZ   4 OZ   5 OZ   6 OZ   7 OZ   8 OZ   9 OZ   10 OZ

TYPE OF EXERCISE/ACTIVITY	HOW LONG?	INTENSITY	CALORIES BURNED
TOTAL CALORIES BURNED:			

SLEEP TRACKER:

◯ ◯ ◯ ◯ ◯ ◯ ◯ ◯ ◯ ◯
1 hr 2 hrs 3 hrs 4 hrs 5 hrs 6 hrs 7 hrs 8 hrs 9 hrs 10 hrs

QUALITY OF SLEEP
☆ ☆ ☆ ☆ ☆

Describe your mood throughout the day. Note in particular the times when you felt 'high' or 'low'. What food/activity affected your mood and/or overall well-being today?

_____

_____

_____

_____

What did you crave today? When did you crave it, and why?
What did you do to manage your cravings throughout the day? Were you successful?

_____

_____

_____

_____

Additional notes/observations i.e. weight, muscle tone, shape, setbacks, motivation etc.

_____

_____

_____

_____

How can you make tomorrow even better?

_____

_____

_____

_____

DAY 31

BREAKFAST	CALORIES	CARBS (g)	FAT (g)	PROTEIN (g)	FIBER (g)	SUGAR (g)	SODIUM (mg)
MORNING SNACK							
TOTAL:							

LUNCH	CALORIES	CARBS (g)	FAT (g)	PROTEIN (g)	FIBER (g)	SUGAR (g)	SODIUM (mg)
MIDDAY SNACK							
TOTAL:							

DINNER	CALORIES	CARBS (g)	FAT (g)	PROTEIN (g)	FIBER (g)	SUGAR (g)	SODIUM (mg)
EVENING SNACK							
TOTAL:							

DAILY TOTAL:

WATER INTAKE:

1 OZ   2 OZ   3 OZ   4 OZ   5 OZ   6 OZ   7 OZ   8 OZ   9 OZ   10 OZ

TYPE OF EXERCISE/ACTIVITY	HOW LONG?	INTENSITY	CALORIES BURNED
		TOTAL CALORIES BURNED:	

SLEEP TRACKER:

○ ○ ○ ○ ○ ○ ○ ○ ○ ○
1 hr   2 hrs   3 hrs   4 hrs   5 hrs   6 hrs   7 hrs   8 hrs   9 hrs   10 hrs

QUALITY OF SLEEP
☆ ☆ ☆ ☆ ☆

Describe your mood throughout the day. Note in particular the times when you felt 'high' or 'low'.
What food/activity affected your mood and/or overall well-being today?

_____

_____

_____

_____

What did you crave today? When did you crave it, and why?
What did you do to manage your cravings throughout the day? Were you successful?

_____

_____

_____

_____

Additional notes/observations i.e. weight, muscle tone, shape, setbacks, motivation etc.

_____

_____

_____

_____

How can you make tomorrow even better?

_____

_____

_____

_____

DAY 32

BREAKFAST	CALORIES	CARBS (g)	FAT (g)	PROTEIN (g)	FIBER (g)	SUGAR (g)	SODIUM (mg)
MORNING SNACK							
TOTAL:							

LUNCH	CALORIES	CARBS (g)	FAT (g)	PROTEIN (g)	FIBER (g)	SUGAR (g)	SODIUM (mg)
MIDDAY SNACK							
TOTAL:							

DINNER	CALORIES	CARBS (g)	FAT (g)	PROTEIN (g)	FIBER (g)	SUGAR (g)	SODIUM (mg)
EVENING SNACK							
TOTAL:							

DAILY TOTAL:

WATER INTAKE:

1 OZ   2 OZ   3 OZ   4 OZ   5 OZ   6 OZ   7 OZ   8 OZ   9 OZ   10 OZ

TYPE OF EXERCISE/ACTIVITY	HOW LONG?	INTENSITY	CALORIES BURNED
TOTAL CALORIES BURNED:			

SLEEP TRACKER:

○ ○ ○ ○ ○ ○ ○ ○ ○ ○
1 hr 2 hrs 3 hrs 4 hrs 5 hrs 6 hrs 7 hrs 8 hrs 9 hrs 10 hrs

QUALITY OF SLEEP
☆ ☆ ☆ ☆ ☆

Describe your mood throughout the day. Note in particular the times when you felt 'high' or 'low'. What food/activity affected your mood and/or overall well-being today?

_____

_____

_____

_____

What did you crave today? When did you crave it, and why?
What did you do to manage your cravings throughout the day? Were you successful?

_____

_____

_____

_____

Additional notes/observations i.e. weight, muscle tone, shape, setbacks, motivation etc.

_____

_____

_____

_____

How can you make tomorrow even better?

_____

_____

_____

_____

DAY 33

BREAKFAST	CALORIES	CARBS (g)	FAT (g)	PROTEIN (g)	FIBER (g)	SUGAR (g)	SODIUM (mg)
MORNING SNACK							
TOTAL:							

LUNCH	CALORIES	CARBS (g)	FAT (g)	PROTEIN (g)	FIBER (g)	SUGAR (g)	SODIUM (mg)
MIDDAY SNACK							
TOTAL:							

DINNER	CALORIES	CARBS (g)	FAT (g)	PROTEIN (g)	FIBER (g)	SUGAR (g)	SODIUM (mg)
EVENING SNACK							
TOTAL:							

DAILY TOTAL:							

WATER INTAKE:

▭ ▭ ▭ ▭ ▭ ▭ ▭ ▭ ▭ ▭
1 OZ 2 OZ 3 OZ 4 OZ 5 OZ 6 OZ 7 OZ 8 OZ 9 OZ 10 OZ

TYPE OF EXERCISE/ACTIVITY	HOW LONG?	INTENSITY	CALORIES BURNED
	TOTAL CALORIES BURNED:		

SLEEP TRACKER:

◯   ◯   ◯   ◯   ◯   ◯   ◯   ◯   ◯   ◯
1 hr   2 hrs   3 hrs   4 hrs   5 hrs   6 hrs   7 hrs   8 hrs   9 hrs   10 hrs

QUALITY OF SLEEP
☆ ☆ ☆ ☆ ☆

Describe your mood throughout the day. Note in particular the times when you felt 'high' or 'low'. What food/activity affected your mood and/or overall well-being today?

_____

_____

_____

_____

What did you crave today? When did you crave it, and why?
What did you do to manage your cravings throughout the day? Were you successful?

_____

_____

_____

_____

Additional notes/observations i.e. weight, muscle tone, shape, setbacks, motivation etc.

_____

_____

_____

How can you make tomorrow even better?

_____

_____

_____

DAY 34

M   T   W   T   F   S   S

DAY: _____   MONTH: _____   YEAR: _____

BREAKFAST	CALORIES	CARBS (g)	FAT (g)	PROTEIN (g)	FIBER (g)	SUGAR (g)	SODIUM (mg)
MORNING SNACK							
TOTAL:							

LUNCH	CALORIES	CARBS (g)	FAT (g)	PROTEIN (g)	FIBER (g)	SUGAR (g)	SODIUM (mg)
MIDDAY SNACK							
TOTAL:							

DINNER	CALORIES	CARBS (g)	FAT (g)	PROTEIN (g)	FIBER (g)	SUGAR (g)	SODIUM (mg)
EVENING SNACK							
TOTAL:							

DAILY TOTAL:

WATER INTAKE:

1 OZ   2 OZ   3 OZ   4 OZ   5 OZ   6 OZ   7 OZ   8 OZ   9 OZ   10 OZ

TYPE OF EXERCISE/ACTIVITY	HOW LONG?	INTENSITY	CALORIES BURNED
TOTAL CALORIES BURNED:			

SLEEP TRACKER:

○ ○ ○ ○ ○ ○ ○ ○ ○ ○
1 hr 2 hrs 3 hrs 4 hrs 5 hrs 6 hrs 7 hrs 8 hrs 9 hrs 10 hrs

QUALITY OF SLEEP
☆ ☆ ☆ ☆ ☆

Describe your mood throughout the day. Note in particular the times when you felt 'high' or 'low'. What food/activity affected your mood and/or overall well-being today?

_____

_____

_____

_____

What did you crave today? When did you crave it, and why?
What did you do to manage your cravings throughout the day? Were you successful?

_____

_____

_____

_____

Additional notes/observations i.e. weight, muscle tone, shape, setbacks, motivation etc.

_____

_____

_____

_____

How can you make tomorrow even better?

_____

_____

_____

_____

DAY 35

M T W T F S S

DAY: _____   MONTH: _____   YEAR: _____

BREAKFAST	CALORIES	CARBS (g)	FAT (g)	PROTEIN (g)	FIBER (g)	SUGAR (g)	SODIUM (mg)
MORNING SNACK							
TOTAL:							

LUNCH	CALORIES	CARBS (g)	FAT (g)	PROTEIN (g)	FIBER (g)	SUGAR (g)	SODIUM (mg)
MIDDAY SNACK							
TOTAL:							

DINNER	CALORIES	CARBS (g)	FAT (g)	PROTEIN (g)	FIBER (g)	SUGAR (g)	SODIUM (mg)
EVENING SNACK							
TOTAL:							

DAILY TOTAL:

WATER INTAKE:

1 OZ   2 OZ   3 OZ   4 OZ   5 OZ   6 OZ   7 OZ   8 OZ   9 OZ   10 OZ

TYPE OF EXERCISE/ACTIVITY	HOW LONG?	INTENSITY	CALORIES BURNED
		TOTAL CALORIES BURNED:	

SLEEP TRACKER:

◯ ◯ ◯ ◯ ◯ ◯ ◯ ◯ ◯ ◯
1 hr   2 hrs   3 hrs   4 hrs   5 hrs   6 hrs   7 hrs   8 hrs   9 hrs   10 hrs

QUALITY OF SLEEP
☆ ☆ ☆ ☆ ☆

Describe your mood throughout the day. Note in particular the times when you felt 'high' or 'low'. What food/activity affected your mood and/or overall well-being today?

_____

_____

_____

_____

What did you crave today? When did you crave it, and why?
What did you do to manage your cravings throughout the day? Were you successful?

_____

_____

_____

_____

Additional notes/observations i.e. weight, muscle tone, shape, setbacks, motivation etc.

_____

_____

_____

_____

How can you make tomorrow even better?

_____

_____

_____

_____

DAY 36

BREAKFAST	CALORIES	CARBS (g)	FAT (g)	PROTEIN (g)	FIBER (g)	SUGAR (g)	SODIUM (mg)
MORNING SNACK							
TOTAL:							

LUNCH	CALORIES	CARBS (g)	FAT (g)	PROTEIN (g)	FIBER (g)	SUGAR (g)	SODIUM (mg)
MIDDAY SNACK							
TOTAL:							

DINNER	CALORIES	CARBS (g)	FAT (g)	PROTEIN (g)	FIBER (g)	SUGAR (g)	SODIUM (mg)
EVENING SNACK							
TOTAL:							

DAILY TOTAL:							

WATER INTAKE:

1 OZ 2 OZ 3 OZ 4 OZ 5 OZ 6 OZ 7 OZ 8 OZ 9 OZ 10 OZ

TYPE OF EXERCISE/ACTIVITY	HOW LONG?	INTENSITY	CALORIES BURNED
	TOTAL CALORIES BURNED:		

SLEEP TRACKER:

◯   ◯   ◯   ◯   ◯   ◯   ◯   ◯   ◯   ◯

1 hr   2 hrs   3 hrs   4 hrs   5 hrs   6 hrs   7 hrs   8 hrs   9 hrs   10 hrs

QUALITY OF SLEEP

☆ ☆ ☆ ☆ ☆

Describe your mood throughout the day. Note in particular the times when you felt 'high' or 'low'. What food/activity affected your mood and/or overall well-being today?

_____

_____

_____

_____

What did you crave today? When did you crave it, and why?
What did you do to manage your cravings throughout the day? Were you successful?

_____

_____

_____

_____

Additional notes/observations i.e. weight, muscle tone, shape, setbacks, motivation etc.

_____

_____

_____

_____

How can you make tomorrow even better?

_____

_____

_____

_____

DAY 37

BREAKFAST	CALORIES	CARBS (g)	FAT (g)	PROTEIN (g)	FIBER (g)	SUGAR (g)	SODIUM (mg)
MORNING SNACK							
TOTAL:							

LUNCH	CALORIES	CARBS (g)	FAT (g)	PROTEIN (g)	FIBER (g)	SUGAR (g)	SODIUM (mg)
MIDDAY SNACK							
TOTAL:							

DINNER	CALORIES	CARBS (g)	FAT (g)	PROTEIN (g)	FIBER (g)	SUGAR (g)	SODIUM (mg)
EVENING SNACK							
TOTAL:							

DAILY TOTAL:							

WATER INTAKE:

1 OZ 2 OZ 3 OZ 4 OZ 5 OZ 6 OZ 7 OZ 8 OZ 9 OZ 10 OZ

TYPE OF EXERCISE/ACTIVITY	HOW LONG?	INTENSITY	CALORIES BURNED
TOTAL CALORIES BURNED:			

SLEEP TRACKER:

◯ ◯ ◯ ◯ ◯ ◯ ◯ ◯ ◯ ◯
1 hr 2 hrs 3 hrs 4 hrs 5 hrs 6 hrs 7 hrs 8 hrs 9 hrs 10 hrs

QUALITY OF SLEEP
☆ ☆ ☆ ☆ ☆

Describe your mood throughout the day. Note in particular the times when you felt 'high' or 'low'.
What food/activity affected your mood and/or overall well-being today?

_____

_____

_____

_____

What did you crave today? When did you crave it, and why?
What did you do to manage your cravings throughout the day? Were you successful?

_____

_____

_____

_____

Additional notes/observations i.e. weight, muscle tone, shape, setbacks, motivation etc.

_____

_____

_____

_____

How can you make tomorrow even better?

_____

_____

_____

_____

DAY 38

M T W T F S S

DAY: _____   MONTH: _____   YEAR: _____

BREAKFAST	CALORIES	CARBS (g)	FAT (g)	PROTEIN (g)	FIBER (g)	SUGAR (g)	SODIUM (mg)
MORNING SNACK							
TOTAL:							

LUNCH	CALORIES	CARBS (g)	FAT (g)	PROTEIN (g)	FIBER (g)	SUGAR (g)	SODIUM (mg)
MIDDAY SNACK							
TOTAL:							

DINNER	CALORIES	CARBS (g)	FAT (g)	PROTEIN (g)	FIBER (g)	SUGAR (g)	SODIUM (mg)
EVENING SNACK							
TOTAL:							

DAILY TOTAL:							

WATER INTAKE:

☐ ☐ ☐ ☐ ☐ ☐ ☐ ☐ ☐ ☐
1 OZ 2 OZ 3 OZ 4 OZ 5 OZ 6 OZ 7 OZ 8 OZ 9 OZ 10 OZ

TYPE OF EXERCISE/ACTIVITY	HOW LONG?	INTENSITY	CALORIES BURNED
		TOTAL CALORIES BURNED:	

SLEEP TRACKER:

◯ ◯ ◯ ◯ ◯ ◯ ◯ ◯ ◯ ◯
1 hr 2 hrs 3 hrs 4 hrs 5 hrs 6 hrs 7 hrs 8 hrs 9 hrs 10 hrs

QUALITY OF SLEEP
☆ ☆ ☆ ☆ ☆

Describe your mood throughout the day. Note in particular the times when you felt 'high' or 'low'. What food/activity affected your mood and/or overall well-being today?

_____
_____
_____
_____

What did you crave today? When did you crave it, and why?
What did you do to manage your cravings throughout the day? Were you successful?

_____
_____
_____
_____

Additional notes/observations i.e. weight, muscle tone, shape, setbacks, motivation etc.

_____
_____
_____
_____

How can you make tomorrow even better?

_____
_____
_____
_____

DAY 39

DAY: _____   MONTH: _____   YEAR: _____

BREAKFAST	CALORIES	CARBS (g)	FAT (g)	PROTEIN (g)	FIBER (g)	SUGAR (g)	SODIUM (mg)
MORNING SNACK							
TOTAL:							

LUNCH	CALORIES	CARBS (g)	FAT (g)	PROTEIN (g)	FIBER (g)	SUGAR (g)	SODIUM (mg)
MIDDAY SNACK							
TOTAL:							

DINNER	CALORIES	CARBS (g)	FAT (g)	PROTEIN (g)	FIBER (g)	SUGAR (g)	SODIUM (mg)
EVENING SNACK							
TOTAL:							

DAILY TOTAL:

WATER INTAKE:

1 OZ 2 OZ 3 OZ 4 OZ 5 OZ 6 OZ 7 OZ 8 OZ 9 OZ 10 OZ

TYPE OF EXERCISE/ACTIVITY	HOW LONG?	INTENSITY	CALORIES BURNED
	TOTAL CALORIES BURNED:		

SLEEP TRACKER:

◯ ◯ ◯ ◯ ◯ ◯ ◯ ◯ ◯ ◯
1 hr 2 hrs 3 hrs 4 hrs 5 hrs 6 hrs 7 hrs 8 hrs 9 hrs 10 hrs

QUALITY OF SLEEP
☆ ☆ ☆ ☆ ☆

Describe your mood throughout the day. Note in particular the times when you felt 'high' or 'low'. What food/activity affected your mood and/or overall well-being today?

_____

_____

_____

_____

What did you crave today? When did you crave it, and why?
What did you do to manage your cravings throughout the day? Were you successful?

_____

_____

_____

_____

Additional notes/observations i.e. weight, muscle tone, shape, setbacks, motivation etc.

_____

_____

_____

_____

How can you make tomorrow even better?

_____

_____

_____

_____

DAY 40

BREAKFAST	CALORIES	CARBS (g)	FAT (g)	PROTEIN (g)	FIBER (g)	SUGAR (g)	SODIUM (mg)
MORNING SNACK							
TOTAL:							

LUNCH	CALORIES	CARBS (g)	FAT (g)	PROTEIN (g)	FIBER (g)	SUGAR (g)	SODIUM (mg)
MIDDAY SNACK							
TOTAL:							

DINNER	CALORIES	CARBS (g)	FAT (g)	PROTEIN (g)	FIBER (g)	SUGAR (g)	SODIUM (mg)
EVENING SNACK							
TOTAL:							
DAILY TOTAL:							

WATER INTAKE:

1 OZ 2 OZ 3 OZ 4 OZ 5 OZ 6 OZ 7 OZ 8 OZ 9 OZ 10 OZ

TYPE OF EXERCISE/ACTIVITY	HOW LONG?	INTENSITY	CALORIES BURNED
	TOTAL CALORIES BURNED:		

SLEEP TRACKER:

◯ ◯ ◯ ◯ ◯ ◯ ◯ ◯ ◯ ◯
1 hr 2 hrs 3 hrs 4 hrs 5 hrs 6 hrs 7 hrs 8 hrs 9 hrs 10 hrs

QUALITY OF SLEEP
☆ ☆ ☆ ☆ ☆

Describe your mood throughout the day. Note in particular the times when you felt 'high' or 'low'. What food/activity affected your mood and/or overall well-being today?

_____

_____

_____

_____

What did you crave today? When did you crave it, and why?
What did you do to manage your cravings throughout the day? Were you successful?

_____

_____

_____

_____

Additional notes/observations i.e. weight, muscle tone, shape, setbacks, motivation etc.

_____

_____

_____

_____

How can you make tomorrow even better?

_____

_____

_____

_____

DAY 41

BREAKFAST	CALORIES	CARBS (g)	FAT (g)	PROTEIN (g)	FIBER (g)	SUGAR (g)	SODIUM (mg)
MORNING SNACK							
TOTAL:							

LUNCH	CALORIES	CARBS (g)	FAT (g)	PROTEIN (g)	FIBER (g)	SUGAR (g)	SODIUM (mg)
MIDDAY SNACK							
TOTAL:							

DINNER	CALORIES	CARBS (g)	FAT (g)	PROTEIN (g)	FIBER (g)	SUGAR (g)	SODIUM (mg)
EVENING SNACK							
TOTAL:							

| DAILY TOTAL: | | | | | | | |

WATER INTAKE:

☐   ☐   ☐   ☐   ☐   ☐   ☐   ☐   ☐   ☐
1 OZ   2 OZ   3 OZ   4 OZ   5 OZ   6 OZ   7 OZ   8 OZ   9 OZ   10 OZ

TYPE OF EXERCISE/ACTIVITY	HOW LONG?	INTENSITY	CALORIES BURNED
		TOTAL CALORIES BURNED:	

SLEEP TRACKER:

○   ○   ○   ○   ○   ○   ○   ○   ○   ○

1 hr   2 hrs   3 hrs   4 hrs   5 hrs   6 hrs   7 hrs   8 hrs   9 hrs   10 hrs

QUALITY OF SLEEP

☆ ☆ ☆ ☆ ☆

Describe your mood throughout the day. Note in particular the times when you felt 'high' or 'low'. What food/activity affected your mood and/or overall well-being today?

_____

_____

_____

_____

What did you crave today? When did you crave it, and why?
What did you do to manage your cravings throughout the day? Were you successful?

_____

_____

_____

_____

Additional notes/observations i.e. weight, muscle tone, shape, setbacks, motivation etc.

_____

_____

_____

How can you make tomorrow even better?

_____

_____

_____

_____

DAY 42

DAY: _____ MONTH: _____ YEAR: _____

BREAKFAST	CALORIES	CARBS (g)	FAT (g)	PROTEIN (g)	FIBER (g)	SUGAR (g)	SODIUM (mg)
MORNING SNACK							
TOTAL:							

LUNCH	CALORIES	CARBS (g)	FAT (g)	PROTEIN (g)	FIBER (g)	SUGAR (g)	SODIUM (mg)
MIDDAY SNACK							
TOTAL:							

DINNER	CALORIES	CARBS (g)	FAT (g)	PROTEIN (g)	FIBER (g)	SUGAR (g)	SODIUM (mg)
EVENING SNACK							
TOTAL:							

DAILY TOTAL:							

WATER INTAKE:

☐ ☐ ☐ ☐ ☐ ☐ ☐ ☐ ☐ ☐
1 OZ 2 OZ 3 OZ 4 OZ 5 OZ 6 OZ 7 OZ 8 OZ 9 OZ 10 OZ

TYPE OF EXERCISE/ACTIVITY	HOW LONG?	INTENSITY	CALORIES BURNED
TOTAL CALORIES BURNED:			

SLEEP TRACKER:

○ ○ ○ ○ ○ ○ ○ ○ ○ ○
1 hr 2 hrs 3 hrs 4 hrs 5 hrs 6 hrs 7 hrs 8 hrs 9 hrs 10 hrs

QUALITY OF SLEEP
☆ ☆ ☆ ☆ ☆

Describe your mood throughout the day. Note in particular the times when you felt 'high' or 'low'. What food/activity affected your mood and/or overall well-being today?

_____

_____

_____

_____

What did you crave today? When did you crave it, and why?
What did you do to manage your cravings throughout the day? Were you successful?

_____

_____

_____

_____

Additional notes/observations i.e. weight, muscle tone, shape, setbacks, motivation etc.

_____

_____

_____

_____

How can you make tomorrow even better?

_____

_____

_____

_____

DAY 43

BREAKFAST	CALORIES	CARBS (g)	FAT (g)	PROTEIN (g)	FIBER (g)	SUGAR (g)	SODIUM (mg)
MORNING SNACK							
TOTAL:							

LUNCH	CALORIES	CARBS (g)	FAT (g)	PROTEIN (g)	FIBER (g)	SUGAR (g)	SODIUM (mg)
MIDDAY SNACK							
TOTAL:							

DINNER	CALORIES	CARBS (g)	FAT (g)	PROTEIN (g)	FIBER (g)	SUGAR (g)	SODIUM (mg)
EVENING SNACK							
TOTAL:							

DAILY TOTAL:							

WATER INTAKE:

1 OZ 2 OZ 3 OZ 4 OZ 5 OZ 6 OZ 7 OZ 8 OZ 9 OZ 10 OZ

TYPE OF EXERCISE/ACTIVITY	HOW LONG?	INTENSITY	CALORIES BURNED
TOTAL CALORIES BURNED:			

SLEEP TRACKER:

◯ ◯ ◯ ◯ ◯ ◯ ◯ ◯ ◯ ◯
1 hr 2 hrs 3 hrs 4 hrs 5 hrs 6 hrs 7 hrs 8 hrs 9 hrs 10 hrs

QUALITY OF SLEEP
☆ ☆ ☆ ☆ ☆

Describe your mood throughout the day. Note in particular the times when you felt 'high' or 'low'.
What food/activity affected your mood and/or overall well-being today?

_____

_____

_____

_____

What did you crave today? When did you crave it, and why?
What did you do to manage your cravings throughout the day? Were you successful?

_____

_____

_____

_____

Additional notes/observations i.e. weight, muscle tone, shape, setbacks, motivation etc.

_____

_____

_____

_____

How can you make tomorrow even better?

_____

_____

_____

_____

DAY 44

M T W T F S S

DAY: _____   MONTH: _____   YEAR: _____

BREAKFAST	CALORIES	CARBS (g)	FAT (g)	PROTEIN (g)	FIBER (g)	SUGAR (g)	SODIUM (mg)
MORNING SNACK							
TOTAL:							

LUNCH	CALORIES	CARBS (g)	FAT (g)	PROTEIN (g)	FIBER (g)	SUGAR (g)	SODIUM (mg)
MIDDAY SNACK							
TOTAL:							

DINNER	CALORIES	CARBS (g)	FAT (g)	PROTEIN (g)	FIBER (g)	SUGAR (g)	SODIUM (mg)
EVENING SNACK							
TOTAL:							

DAILY TOTAL:

WATER INTAKE:

1 OZ   2 OZ   3 OZ   4 OZ   5 OZ   6 OZ   7 OZ   8 OZ   9 OZ   10 OZ

TYPE OF EXERCISE/ACTIVITY	HOW LONG?	INTENSITY	CALORIES BURNED
TOTAL CALORIES BURNED:			

SLEEP TRACKER:

○ ○ ○ ○ ○ ○ ○ ○ ○ ○
1 hr   2 hrs   3 hrs   4 hrs   5 hrs   6 hrs   7 hrs   8 hrs   9 hrs   10 hrs

QUALITY OF SLEEP
☆ ☆ ☆ ☆ ☆

Describe your mood throughout the day. Note in particular the times when you felt 'high' or 'low'. What food/activity affected your mood and/or overall well-being today?

_____

_____

_____

_____

What did you crave today? When did you crave it, and why?
What did you do to manage your cravings throughout the day? Were you successful?

_____

_____

_____

_____

Additional notes/observations i.e. weight, muscle tone, shape, setbacks, motivation etc.

_____

_____

_____

_____

How can you make tomorrow even better?

_____

_____

_____

_____

DAY 45

M T W T F S S

DAY: _____   MONTH: _____   YEAR: _____

BREAKFAST	CALORIES	CARBS (g)	FAT (g)	PROTEIN (g)	FIBER (g)	SUGAR (g)	SODIUM (mg)
MORNING SNACK							
TOTAL:							

LUNCH	CALORIES	CARBS (g)	FAT (g)	PROTEIN (g)	FIBER (g)	SUGAR (g)	SODIUM (mg)
MIDDAY SNACK							
TOTAL:							

DINNER	CALORIES	CARBS (g)	FAT (g)	PROTEIN (g)	FIBER (g)	SUGAR (g)	SODIUM (mg)
EVENING SNACK							
TOTAL:							

| DAILY TOTAL: | | | | | | | |

WATER INTAKE:

☐ ☐ ☐ ☐ ☐ ☐ ☐ ☐ ☐ ☐
1 OZ 2 OZ 3 OZ 4 OZ 5 OZ 6 OZ 7 OZ 8 OZ 9 OZ 10 OZ

TYPE OF EXERCISE/ACTIVITY	HOW LONG?	INTENSITY	CALORIES BURNED
	TOTAL CALORIES BURNED:		

SLEEP TRACKER:

◯ ◯ ◯ ◯ ◯ ◯ ◯ ◯ ◯ ◯
1 hr   2 hrs   3 hrs   4 hrs   5 hrs   6 hrs   7 hrs   8 hrs   9 hrs   10 hrs

QUALITY OF SLEEP
☆ ☆ ☆ ☆ ☆

Describe your mood throughout the day. Note in particular the times when you felt 'high' or 'low'. What food/activity affected your mood and/or overall well-being today?

_____
_____
_____
_____

What did you crave today? When did you crave it, and why?
What did you do to manage your cravings throughout the day? Were you successful?

_____
_____
_____
_____

Additional notes/observations i.e. weight, muscle tone, shape, setbacks, motivation etc.

_____
_____
_____
_____

How can you make tomorrow even better?

_____
_____
_____
_____

DAY 46

DAY: _____   MONTH: _____   YEAR: _____

BREAKFAST	CALORIES	CARBS (g)	FAT (g)	PROTEIN (g)	FIBER (g)	SUGAR (g)	SODIUM (mg)
MORNING SNACK							
TOTAL:							

LUNCH	CALORIES	CARBS (g)	FAT (g)	PROTEIN (g)	FIBER (g)	SUGAR (g)	SODIUM (mg)
MIDDAY SNACK							
TOTAL:							

DINNER	CALORIES	CARBS (g)	FAT (g)	PROTEIN (g)	FIBER (g)	SUGAR (g)	SODIUM (mg)
EVENING SNACK							
TOTAL:							

DAILY TOTAL:

WATER INTAKE:

1 OZ   2 OZ   3 OZ   4 OZ   5 OZ   6 OZ   7 OZ   8 OZ   9 OZ   10 OZ

TYPE OF EXERCISE/ACTIVITY	HOW LONG?	INTENSITY	CALORIES BURNED
TOTAL CALORIES BURNED:			

SLEEP TRACKER:

○ ○ ○ ○ ○ ○ ○ ○ ○ ○
1 hr 2 hrs 3 hrs 4 hrs 5 hrs 6 hrs 7 hrs 8 hrs 9 hrs 10 hrs

QUALITY OF SLEEP
☆ ☆ ☆ ☆ ☆

Describe your mood throughout the day. Note in particular the times when you felt 'high' or 'low'. What food/activity affected your mood and/or overall well-being today?

_____

_____

_____

_____

What did you crave today? When did you crave it, and why?
What did you do to manage your cravings throughout the day? Were you successful?

_____

_____

_____

_____

Additional notes/observations i.e. weight, muscle tone, shape, setbacks, motivation etc.

_____

_____

_____

_____

How can you make tomorrow even better?

_____

_____

_____

_____

DAY 47

BREAKFAST	CALORIES	CARBS (g)	FAT (g)	PROTEIN (g)	FIBER (g)	SUGAR (g)	SODIUM (mg)
MORNING SNACK							
TOTAL:							

LUNCH	CALORIES	CARBS (g)	FAT (g)	PROTEIN (g)	FIBER (g)	SUGAR (g)	SODIUM (mg)
MIDDAY SNACK							
TOTAL:							

DINNER	CALORIES	CARBS (g)	FAT (g)	PROTEIN (g)	FIBER (g)	SUGAR (g)	SODIUM (mg)
EVENING SNACK							
TOTAL:							

DAILY TOTAL:

WATER INTAKE:

☐ ☐ ☐ ☐ ☐ ☐ ☐ ☐ ☐ ☐
1 OZ 2 OZ 3 OZ 4 OZ 5 OZ 6 OZ 7 OZ 8 OZ 9 OZ 10 OZ

TYPE OF EXERCISE/ACTIVITY	HOW LONG?	INTENSITY	CALORIES BURNED
TOTAL CALORIES BURNED:			

SLEEP TRACKER:

○ ○ ○ ○ ○ ○ ○ ○ ○ ○
1 hr 2 hrs 3 hrs 4 hrs 5 hrs 6 hrs 7 hrs 8 hrs 9 hrs 10 hrs

QUALITY OF SLEEP
☆ ☆ ☆ ☆ ☆

Describe your mood throughout the day. Note in particular the times when you felt 'high' or 'low'. What food/activity affected your mood and/or overall well-being today?

_____

_____

_____

_____

What did you crave today? When did you crave it, and why?
What did you do to manage your cravings throughout the day? Were you successful?

_____

_____

_____

_____

Additional notes/observations i.e. weight, muscle tone, shape, setbacks, motivation etc.

_____

_____

_____

_____

How can you make tomorrow even better?

_____

_____

_____

_____

DAY 48

BREAKFAST	CALORIES	CARBS (g)	FAT (g)	PROTEIN (g)	FIBER (g)	SUGAR (g)	SODIUM (mg)
MORNING SNACK							
TOTAL:							

LUNCH	CALORIES	CARBS (g)	FAT (g)	PROTEIN (g)	FIBER (g)	SUGAR (g)	SODIUM (mg)
MIDDAY SNACK							
TOTAL:							

DINNER	CALORIES	CARBS (g)	FAT (g)	PROTEIN (g)	FIBER (g)	SUGAR (g)	SODIUM (mg)
EVENING SNACK							
TOTAL:							

DAILY TOTAL:							

WATER INTAKE:

1 OZ 2 OZ 3 OZ 4 OZ 5 OZ 6 OZ 7 OZ 8 OZ 9 OZ 10 OZ

TYPE OF EXERCISE/ACTIVITY	HOW LONG?	INTENSITY	CALORIES BURNED
TOTAL CALORIES BURNED:			

SLEEP TRACKER:

○ ○ ○ ○ ○ ○ ○ ○ ○ ○
1 hr 2 hrs 3 hrs 4 hrs 5 hrs 6 hrs 7 hrs 8 hrs 9 hrs 10 hrs

QUALITY OF SLEEP
☆ ☆ ☆ ☆ ☆

Describe your mood throughout the day. Note in particular the times when you felt 'high' or 'low'. What food/activity affected your mood and/or overall well-being today?

_____

_____

_____

What did you crave today? When did you crave it, and why?
What did you do to manage your cravings throughout the day? Were you successful?

_____

_____

_____

Additional notes/observations i.e. weight, muscle tone, shape, setbacks, motivation etc.

_____

_____

_____

How can you make tomorrow even better?

_____

_____

_____

DAY 49

DAY: _____ MONTH: _____ YEAR: _____

BREAKFAST	CALORIES	CARBS (g)	FAT (g)	PROTEIN (g)	FIBER (g)	SUGAR (g)	SODIUM (mg)
MORNING SNACK							
TOTAL:							

LUNCH	CALORIES	CARBS (g)	FAT (g)	PROTEIN (g)	FIBER (g)	SUGAR (g)	SODIUM (mg)
MIDDAY SNACK							
TOTAL:							

DINNER	CALORIES	CARBS (g)	FAT (g)	PROTEIN (g)	FIBER (g)	SUGAR (g)	SODIUM (mg)
EVENING SNACK							
TOTAL:							

DAILY TOTAL:							

WATER INTAKE:

1 OZ 2 OZ 3 OZ 4 OZ 5 OZ 6 OZ 7 OZ 8 OZ 9 OZ 10 OZ

TYPE OF EXERCISE/ACTIVITY	HOW LONG?	INTENSITY	CALORIES BURNED
	TOTAL CALORIES BURNED:		

SLEEP TRACKER:

○ ○ ○ ○ ○ ○ ○ ○ ○ ○
1 hr   2 hrs   3 hrs   4 hrs   5 hrs   6 hrs   7 hrs   8 hrs   9 hrs   10 hrs

QUALITY OF SLEEP
☆ ☆ ☆ ☆ ☆

Describe your mood throughout the day. Note in particular the times when you felt 'high' or 'low'. What food/activity affected your mood and/or overall well-being today?

_____

_____

_____

_____

What did you crave today? When did you crave it, and why?
What did you do to manage your cravings throughout the day? Were you successful?

_____

_____

_____

_____

Additional notes/observations i.e. weight, muscle tone, shape, setbacks, motivation etc.

_____

_____

_____

_____

How can you make tomorrow even better?

_____

_____

_____

_____

DAY 50

BREAKFAST	CALORIES	CARBS (g)	FAT (g)	PROTEIN (g)	FIBER (g)	SUGAR (g)	SODIUM (mg)
MORNING SNACK							
TOTAL:							

LUNCH	CALORIES	CARBS (g)	FAT (g)	PROTEIN (g)	FIBER (g)	SUGAR (g)	SODIUM (mg)
MIDDAY SNACK							
TOTAL:							

DINNER	CALORIES	CARBS (g)	FAT (g)	PROTEIN (g)	FIBER (g)	SUGAR (g)	SODIUM (mg)
EVENING SNACK							
TOTAL:							

DAILY TOTAL:

WATER INTAKE:

1 OZ   2 OZ   3 OZ   4 OZ   5 OZ   6 OZ   7 OZ   8 OZ   9 OZ   10 OZ

TYPE OF EXERCISE/ACTIVITY	HOW LONG?	INTENSITY	CALORIES BURNED
	TOTAL CALORIES BURNED:		

SLEEP TRACKER:

○ ○ ○ ○ ○ ○ ○ ○ ○ ○
1 hr   2 hrs   3 hrs   4 hrs   5 hrs   6 hrs   7 hrs   8 hrs   9 hrs   10 hrs

QUALITY OF SLEEP
☆ ☆ ☆ ☆ ☆

Describe your mood throughout the day. Note in particular the times when you felt 'high' or 'low'. What food/activity affected your mood and/or overall well-being today?

_____
_____
_____
_____

What did you crave today? When did you crave it, and why?
What did you do to manage your cravings throughout the day? Were you successful?

_____
_____
_____
_____

Additional notes/observations i.e. weight, muscle tone, shape, setbacks, motivation etc.

_____
_____
_____
_____

How can you make tomorrow even better?

_____
_____
_____
_____

DAY 51

DAY: _____   MONTH: _____   YEAR: _____

BREAKFAST	CALORIES	CARBS (g)	FAT (g)	PROTEIN (g)	FIBER (g)	SUGAR (g)	SODIUM (mg)
MORNING SNACK							
TOTAL:							

LUNCH	CALORIES	CARBS (g)	FAT (g)	PROTEIN (g)	FIBER (g)	SUGAR (g)	SODIUM (mg)
MIDDAY SNACK							
TOTAL:							

DINNER	CALORIES	CARBS (g)	FAT (g)	PROTEIN (g)	FIBER (g)	SUGAR (g)	SODIUM (mg)
EVENING SNACK							
TOTAL:							

DAILY TOTAL:

WATER INTAKE:

1 OZ   2 OZ   3 OZ   4 OZ   5 OZ   6 OZ   7 OZ   8 OZ   9 OZ   10 OZ

TYPE OF EXERCISE/ACTIVITY	HOW LONG?	INTENSITY	CALORIES BURNED
TOTAL CALORIES BURNED:			

SLEEP TRACKER:

○ ○ ○ ○ ○ ○ ○ ○ ○ ○
1 hr　2 hrs　3 hrs　4 hrs　5 hrs　6 hrs　7 hrs　8 hrs　9 hrs　10 hrs

QUALITY OF SLEEP
☆ ☆ ☆ ☆ ☆

Describe your mood throughout the day. Note in particular the times when you felt 'high' or 'low'. What food/activity affected your mood and/or overall well-being today?

_____

_____

_____

_____

What did you crave today? When did you crave it, and why?
What did you do to manage your cravings throughout the day? Were you successful?

_____

_____

_____

_____

Additional notes/observations i.e. weight, muscle tone, shape, setbacks, motivation etc.

_____

_____

_____

_____

How can you make tomorrow even better?

_____

_____

_____

_____

DAY 52

BREAKFAST	CALORIES	CARBS (g)	FAT (g)	PROTEIN (g)	FIBER (g)	SUGAR (g)	SODIUM (mg)
MORNING SNACK							
TOTAL:							

LUNCH	CALORIES	CARBS (g)	FAT (g)	PROTEIN (g)	FIBER (g)	SUGAR (g)	SODIUM (mg)
MIDDAY SNACK							
TOTAL:							

DINNER	CALORIES	CARBS (g)	FAT (g)	PROTEIN (g)	FIBER (g)	SUGAR (g)	SODIUM (mg)
EVENING SNACK							
TOTAL:							
DAILY TOTAL:							

WATER INTAKE:

☐ ☐ ☐ ☐ ☐ ☐ ☐ ☐ ☐ ☐
1 OZ 2 OZ 3 OZ 4 OZ 5 OZ 6 OZ 7 OZ 8 OZ 9 OZ 10 OZ

TYPE OF EXERCISE/ACTIVITY	HOW LONG?	INTENSITY	CALORIES BURNED
	TOTAL CALORIES BURNED:		

SLEEP TRACKER:

○ ○ ○ ○ ○ ○ ○ ○ ○ ○
1 hr 2 hrs 3 hrs 4 hrs 5 hrs 6 hrs 7 hrs 8 hrs 9 hrs 10 hrs

QUALITY OF SLEEP
☆ ☆ ☆ ☆ ☆

Describe your mood throughout the day. Note in particular the times when you felt 'high' or 'low'. What food/activity affected your mood and/or overall well-being today?

_____

_____

_____

What did you crave today? When did you crave it, and why?
What did you do to manage your cravings throughout the day? Were you successful?

_____

_____

_____

Additional notes/observations i.e. weight, muscle tone, shape, setbacks, motivation etc.

_____

_____

_____

How can you make tomorrow even better?

_____

_____

_____

DAY 53

DAY: _____ MONTH: _____ YEAR: _____

BREAKFAST	CALORIES	CARBS (g)	FAT (g)	PROTEIN (g)	FIBER (g)	SUGAR (g)	SODIUM (mg)
MORNING SNACK							
TOTAL:							

LUNCH	CALORIES	CARBS (g)	FAT (g)	PROTEIN (g)	FIBER (g)	SUGAR (g)	SODIUM (mg)
MIDDAY SNACK							
TOTAL:							

DINNER	CALORIES	CARBS (g)	FAT (g)	PROTEIN (g)	FIBER (g)	SUGAR (g)	SODIUM (mg)
EVENING SNACK							
TOTAL:							

DAILY TOTAL:

WATER INTAKE:

☐ ☐ ☐ ☐ ☐ ☐ ☐ ☐ ☐ ☐
1 OZ 2 OZ 3 OZ 4 OZ 5 OZ 6 OZ 7 OZ 8 OZ 9 OZ 10 OZ

TYPE OF EXERCISE/ACTIVITY	HOW LONG?	INTENSITY	CALORIES BURNED
TOTAL CALORIES BURNED:			

SLEEP TRACKER:

○ ○ ○ ○ ○ ○ ○ ○ ○ ○
1 hr 2 hrs 3 hrs 4 hrs 5 hrs 6 hrs 7 hrs 8 hrs 9 hrs 10 hrs

QUALITY OF SLEEP
☆ ☆ ☆ ☆ ☆

Describe your mood throughout the day. Note in particular the times when you felt 'high' or 'low'. What food/activity affected your mood and/or overall well-being today?

_____

_____

_____

_____

What did you crave today? When did you crave it, and why?
What did you do to manage your cravings throughout the day? Were you successful?

_____

_____

_____

_____

Additional notes/observations i.e. weight, muscle tone, shape, setbacks, motivation etc.

_____

_____

_____

_____

How can you make tomorrow even better?

_____

_____

_____

_____

DAY 54

M T W T F S S

DAY: _____ MONTH: _____ YEAR: _____

BREAKFAST	CALORIES	CARBS (g)	FAT (g)	PROTEIN (g)	FIBER (g)	SUGAR (g)	SODIUM (mg)
MORNING SNACK							
TOTAL:							

LUNCH	CALORIES	CARBS (g)	FAT (g)	PROTEIN (g)	FIBER (g)	SUGAR (g)	SODIUM (mg)
MIDDAY SNACK							
TOTAL:							

DINNER	CALORIES	CARBS (g)	FAT (g)	PROTEIN (g)	FIBER (g)	SUGAR (g)	SODIUM (mg)
EVENING SNACK							
TOTAL:							

DAILY TOTAL:							

WATER INTAKE:

⬜ ⬜ ⬜ ⬜ ⬜ ⬜ ⬜ ⬜ ⬜ ⬜
1 OZ 2 OZ 3 OZ 4 OZ 5 OZ 6 OZ 7 OZ 8 OZ 9 OZ 10 OZ

TYPE OF EXERCISE/ACTIVITY	HOW LONG?	INTENSITY	CALORIES BURNED
TOTAL CALORIES BURNED:			

SLEEP TRACKER:

○   ○   ○   ○   ○   ○   ○   ○   ○   ○
1 hr   2 hrs   3 hrs   4 hrs   5 hrs   6 hrs   7 hrs   8 hrs   9 hrs   10 hrs

QUALITY OF SLEEP
☆ ☆ ☆ ☆ ☆

Describe your mood throughout the day. Note in particular the times when you felt 'high' or 'low'. What food/activity affected your mood and/or overall well-being today?

_____

_____

_____

_____

What did you crave today? When did you crave it, and why?
What did you do to manage your cravings throughout the day? Were you successful?

_____

_____

_____

_____

Additional notes/observations i.e. weight, muscle tone, shape, setbacks, motivation etc.

_____

_____

_____

_____

How can you make tomorrow even better?

_____

_____

_____

_____

DAY 55

DAY: _____ MONTH: _____ YEAR: _____

BREAKFAST	CALORIES	CARBS (g)	FAT (g)	PROTEIN (g)	FIBER (g)	SUGAR (g)	SODIUM (mg)
MORNING SNACK							
TOTAL:							

LUNCH	CALORIES	CARBS (g)	FAT (g)	PROTEIN (g)	FIBER (g)	SUGAR (g)	SODIUM (mg)
MIDDAY SNACK							
TOTAL:							

DINNER	CALORIES	CARBS (g)	FAT (g)	PROTEIN (g)	FIBER (g)	SUGAR (g)	SODIUM (mg)
EVENING SNACK							
TOTAL:							

DAILY TOTAL:							

WATER INTAKE:

☐ ☐ ☐ ☐ ☐ ☐ ☐ ☐ ☐ ☐
1 OZ 2 OZ 3 OZ 4 OZ 5 OZ 6 OZ 7 OZ 8 OZ 9 OZ 10 OZ

TYPE OF EXERCISE/ACTIVITY	HOW LONG?	INTENSITY	CALORIES BURNED
TOTAL CALORIES BURNED:			

SLEEP TRACKER:

○ ○ ○ ○ ○ ○ ○ ○ ○ ○
1 hr   2 hrs   3 hrs   4 hrs   5 hrs   6 hrs   7 hrs   8 hrs   9 hrs   10 hrs

QUALITY OF SLEEP
☆ ☆ ☆ ☆ ☆

Describe your mood throughout the day. Note in particular the times when you felt 'high' or 'low'. What food/activity affected your mood and/or overall well-being today?

_____

_____

_____

_____

What did you crave today? When did you crave it, and why?
What did you do to manage your cravings throughout the day? Were you successful?

_____

_____

_____

_____

Additional notes/observations i.e. weight, muscle tone, shape, setbacks, motivation etc.

_____

_____

_____

_____

How can you make tomorrow even better?

_____

_____

_____

_____

DAY 56

BREAKFAST	CALORIES	CARBS (g)	FAT (g)	PROTEIN (g)	FIBER (g)	SUGAR (g)	SODIUM (mg)
MORNING SNACK							
TOTAL:							

LUNCH	CALORIES	CARBS (g)	FAT (g)	PROTEIN (g)	FIBER (g)	SUGAR (g)	SODIUM (mg)
MIDDAY SNACK							
TOTAL:							

DINNER	CALORIES	CARBS (g)	FAT (g)	PROTEIN (g)	FIBER (g)	SUGAR (g)	SODIUM (mg)
EVENING SNACK							
TOTAL:							

DAILY TOTAL:							

WATER INTAKE:

⊔ ⊔ ⊔ ⊔ ⊔ ⊔ ⊔ ⊔ ⊔ ⊔
1 OZ 2 OZ 3 OZ 4 OZ 5 OZ 6 OZ 7 OZ 8 OZ 9 OZ 10 OZ

TYPE OF EXERCISE/ACTIVITY	HOW LONG?	INTENSITY	CALORIES BURNED
TOTAL CALORIES BURNED:			

SLEEP TRACKER:

○ ○ ○ ○ ○ ○ ○ ○ ○ ○
1 hr 2 hrs 3 hrs 4 hrs 5 hrs 6 hrs 7 hrs 8 hrs 9 hrs 10 hrs

QUALITY OF SLEEP
☆ ☆ ☆ ☆ ☆

Describe your mood throughout the day. Note in particular the times when you felt 'high' or 'low'. What food/activity affected your mood and/or overall well-being today?

_____

_____

_____

_____

What did you crave today? When did you crave it, and why?
What did you do to manage your cravings throughout the day? Were you successful?

_____

_____

_____

_____

Additional notes/observations i.e. weight, muscle tone, shape, setbacks, motivation etc.

_____

_____

_____

_____

How can you make tomorrow even better?

_____

_____

_____

_____

DAY 57

DAY: _____ MONTH: _____ YEAR: _____

BREAKFAST	CALORIES	CARBS (g)	FAT (g)	PROTEIN (g)	FIBER (g)	SUGAR (g)	SODIUM (mg)
MORNING SNACK							
TOTAL:							

LUNCH	CALORIES	CARBS (g)	FAT (g)	PROTEIN (g)	FIBER (g)	SUGAR (g)	SODIUM (mg)
MIDDAY SNACK							
TOTAL:							

DINNER	CALORIES	CARBS (g)	FAT (g)	PROTEIN (g)	FIBER (g)	SUGAR (g)	SODIUM (mg)
EVENING SNACK							
TOTAL:							

DAILY TOTAL:

WATER INTAKE:

1 OZ 2 OZ 3 OZ 4 OZ 5 OZ 6 OZ 7 OZ 8 OZ 9 OZ 10 OZ

TYPE OF EXERCISE/ACTIVITY	HOW LONG?	INTENSITY	CALORIES BURNED
		TOTAL CALORIES BURNED:	

SLEEP TRACKER:

◯ ◯ ◯ ◯ ◯ ◯ ◯ ◯ ◯ ◯
1 hr 2 hrs 3 hrs 4 hrs 5 hrs 6 hrs 7 hrs 8 hrs 9 hrs 10 hrs

QUALITY OF SLEEP
☆ ☆ ☆ ☆ ☆

Describe your mood throughout the day. Note in particular the times when you felt 'high' or 'low'. What food/activity affected your mood and/or overall well-being today?

_____

_____

_____

_____

What did you crave today? When did you crave it, and why?
What did you do to manage your cravings throughout the day? Were you successful?

_____

_____

_____

_____

Additional notes/observations i.e. weight, muscle tone, shape, setbacks, motivation etc.

_____

_____

_____

_____

How can you make tomorrow even better?

_____

_____

_____

_____

DAY 58

BREAKFAST	CALORIES	CARBS (g)	FAT (g)	PROTEIN (g)	FIBER (g)	SUGAR (g)	SODIUM (mg)
MORNING SNACK							
TOTAL:							

LUNCH	CALORIES	CARBS (g)	FAT (g)	PROTEIN (g)	FIBER (g)	SUGAR (g)	SODIUM (mg)
MIDDAY SNACK							
TOTAL:							

DINNER	CALORIES	CARBS (g)	FAT (g)	PROTEIN (g)	FIBER (g)	SUGAR (g)	SODIUM (mg)
EVENING SNACK							
TOTAL:							

| **DAILY TOTAL:** | | | | | | | |

WATER INTAKE:

1 OZ   2 OZ   3 OZ   4 OZ   5 OZ   6 OZ   7 OZ   8 OZ   9 OZ   10 OZ

TYPE OF EXERCISE/ACTIVITY	HOW LONG?	INTENSITY	CALORIES BURNED
TOTAL CALORIES BURNED:			

SLEEP TRACKER:

○ ○ ○ ○ ○ ○ ○ ○ ○ ○
1 hr 2 hrs 3 hrs 4 hrs 5 hrs 6 hrs 7 hrs 8 hrs 9 hrs 10 hrs

QUALITY OF SLEEP
☆ ☆ ☆ ☆ ☆

Describe your mood throughout the day. Note in particular the times when you felt 'high' or 'low'. What food/activity affected your mood and/or overall well-being today?

_____

_____

_____

_____

What did you crave today? When did you crave it, and why?
What did you do to manage your cravings throughout the day? Were you successful?

_____

_____

_____

_____

Additional notes/observations i.e. weight, muscle tone, shape, setbacks, motivation etc.

_____

_____

_____

_____

How can you make tomorrow even better?

_____

_____

_____

_____

DAY 59

DAY: _____   MONTH: _____   YEAR: _____

BREAKFAST	CALORIES	CARBS (g)	FAT (g)	PROTEIN (g)	FIBER (g)	SUGAR (g)	SODIUM (mg)
MORNING SNACK							
TOTAL:							

LUNCH	CALORIES	CARBS (g)	FAT (g)	PROTEIN (g)	FIBER (g)	SUGAR (g)	SODIUM (mg)
MIDDAY SNACK							
TOTAL:							

DINNER	CALORIES	CARBS (g)	FAT (g)	PROTEIN (g)	FIBER (g)	SUGAR (g)	SODIUM (mg)
EVENING SNACK							
TOTAL:							

| DAILY TOTAL: | | | | | | | |

WATER INTAKE:

1 OZ   2 OZ   3 OZ   4 OZ   5 OZ   6 OZ   7 OZ   8 OZ   9 OZ   10 OZ

TYPE OF EXERCISE/ACTIVITY	HOW LONG?	INTENSITY	CALORIES BURNED
	TOTAL CALORIES BURNED:		

SLEEP TRACKER:

○ ○ ○ ○ ○ ○ ○ ○ ○ ○
1 hr 2 hrs 3 hrs 4 hrs 5 hrs 6 hrs 7 hrs 8 hrs 9 hrs 10 hrs

QUALITY OF SLEEP
☆ ☆ ☆ ☆ ☆

Describe your mood throughout the day. Note in particular the times when you felt 'high' or 'low'. What food/activity affected your mood and/or overall well-being today?

_____

_____

_____

_____

What did you crave today? When did you crave it, and why?
What did you do to manage your cravings throughout the day? Were you successful?

_____

_____

_____

_____

Additional notes/observations i.e. weight, muscle tone, shape, setbacks, motivation etc.

_____

_____

_____

_____

How can you make tomorrow even better?

_____

_____

_____

_____

DAY 60

BREAKFAST	CALORIES	CARBS (g)	FAT (g)	PROTEIN (g)	FIBER (g)	SUGAR (g)	SODIUM (mg)
MORNING SNACK							
TOTAL:							

LUNCH	CALORIES	CARBS (g)	FAT (g)	PROTEIN (g)	FIBER (g)	SUGAR (g)	SODIUM (mg)
MIDDAY SNACK							
TOTAL:							

DINNER	CALORIES	CARBS (g)	FAT (g)	PROTEIN (g)	FIBER (g)	SUGAR (g)	SODIUM (mg)
EVENING SNACK							
TOTAL:							

DAILY TOTAL:							

WATER INTAKE:

1 OZ   2 OZ   3 OZ   4 OZ   5 OZ   6 OZ   7 OZ   8 OZ   9 OZ   10 OZ

TYPE OF EXERCISE/ACTIVITY	HOW LONG?	INTENSITY	CALORIES BURNED
TOTAL CALORIES BURNED:			

SLEEP TRACKER:

◯   ◯   ◯   ◯   ◯   ◯   ◯   ◯   ◯   ◯

1 hr   2 hrs   3 hrs   4 hrs   5 hrs   6 hrs   7 hrs   8 hrs   9 hrs   10 hrs

QUALITY OF SLEEP

☆ ☆ ☆ ☆ ☆

Describe your mood throughout the day. Note in particular the times when you felt 'high' or 'low'. What food/activity affected your mood and/or overall well-being today?

_____

_____

_____

_____

What did you crave today? When did you crave it, and why?
What did you do to manage your cravings throughout the day? Were you successful?

_____

_____

_____

_____

Additional notes/observations i.e. weight, muscle tone, shape, setbacks, motivation etc.

_____

_____

_____

_____

How can you make tomorrow even better?

_____

_____

_____

_____

Made in the USA
Middletown, DE
10 March 2023

26541337R00071